CHILDBIRTH IN THE GHETTO: FOLK BELIEFS OF NEGRO WOMEN IN A NORTH PHILADELPHIA HOSPITAL WARD

By: BARBARA FRANKEL

San Francisco, California
1977

Published By

R & E Research Associates, Inc.
4843 Mission Street
San Francisco, California 94112

Publishers
Robert D. Reed and Adam S. Eterovich

Library of Congress Card Catalog Number
76-27000

I.S.B.N.
0-88247-418-9

PREFACE

The field work for Childbirth in the Ghetto was carried out in the latter half of 1968 and the early months of 1969. In the few years since that time several things have happened in U. S. society which, if they have not already revolutionized feminine consciousness and behavior, bode fair to do so before much more time has passed. The first of these things was a discrete event: the 1973 Supreme Court decision concerning abortion. This decision invalidated the anti-abortion laws of many states, including Pennsylvania, where my study was carried out. It is now possible for a woman living in the State of Pennsylvania to obtain a safe, legal abortion without the need for the consent of others in her family, and without the need to demonstrate that a full-term pregnancy would place either her mental or physical health at risk. Since 1973 a number of hospitals and clinics in the Philadelphia area have established facilities for routine abortion services to be offered to those wishing to use them.

The second event -- perhaps more aptly called a trend -- is the gradual intensification of vocal public support for antinatalist political and social opinions. Such positions are supported by major segments of the rejuvenated feminist movement, and also by many members of the ecology movement who campaign for "zero population growth." Each of these groups for its own reasons deplores traditional attitudes which make childbearing the supreme validation of the feminine self. Feminists have periodically mounted campaigns which appeal to women to refuse to allow themselves to be defined as "baby machines," while ecologists have pleaded with persons of both sexes to demonstrate social conscience by limiting the number of their offspring.

Neither of these positions would be viable as a real alternative for people were it not for the combined effects of the court decision already mentioned and, even more important, the technology of contraception. This, one gathers, will soon become nearly foolproof with the marketing of a "morning after pill." For the first time in human history it has become possible for women in this and other technologically sophisticated countries to exercise full control over their own procreative potentialities.

At the time my study was carried out, the revolutionary impact of these developments was only beginning to become apparent. Contraceptive devices and information had only recently been made available to women in the Philadelphia ghetto population. Although the trusty diaphragm had been available to middle- and upper-class women for forty or fifty years through their private physicians, and "the Pill" and the intrauterine device (IUD) for perhaps a decade, Public Assistance laws in Pennsylvania and many other states had forbidden them to most clinic patients. Temple University Health Sciences Center, where my field work was carried out, a regular program of birth control education had been put into effect only about two years prior to my arrival.

For me, then, one of the most interesting features of the ghetto folklore I was collecting was the fact that the topic of contraception had already given rise to a rich vein of folklore. The rapidity with which information about "the Pill" and "the coil" had become assimilated to those traditional forms of stereotyped communication generally labeled "beliefs and superstitions" was quite remarkable. Indeed, the speed and thoroughness with which this process occurred supported my contention that "Folklore" is not merely a collection of curios, static and frozen survivals from the past, but rather a living process whereby human beings transmit knowledge to one another in readily memorable form.

I would give a good deal to be able to interview my ghetto informants today in order to find out what new information has been fed into the folkloric communication system since the end of my original study. I suspect that there must be quite a few changes, in view of the dramatic drop in the U. S. birth rate since that time. The media and other sources inform us that the United States is now within hailing distance of "zero population growth" -- with the sharpest drop of all among the lower classes, to whom planned parenthood is a relative novelty.

If it were possible to interview the same informants today, I would expect the greatest alterations in knowledge and belief to be found in connection with one subject: abortion. At the time of my study this was still a topic surrounded by strong tabus, such that my informants rarely mentioned it spontaneously or discussed it willingly. Those who did so always denied having attempted to seek abortions themselves at any time, and the folklore on the subject was fraught with overtones of fear and moral disapproval. The illegality of abortion in 1968 made it dangerous both socially and physically, of course; but in addition ghetto women saw it as wrong, and tended to view the dangers of abortion as moral judgements visited upon women who lacked proper maternal feeling.

At the same time, however, there were innumerable hints of individual desperation and despair as older women faced the prospect of another mouth to feed, and young girls the prospect of youth and education cut short by pregnancies that were most often out of wedlock. If, as I suspect, the legalization of abortion has freed large numbers of such women from the physical and legal jeopardy that once attended efforts to terminate unwanted pregnancy, I think it plausible to suppose that much of the moral disapproval has been dissipated along with the danger.

On the other hand I would not really expect so radical a transformation that women no longer desire children as validation of their femininity, as objects of affection, as extensions of themselves and their husbands, as a form of social security -- or for any of the other reasons for which human beings have wanted and welcomed offspring since time immemorial. Indeed, I would suppose -- recalling the plucky independence which many ghetto women exhibited in regard to the trendy ideologies of the upper classes -- that antinatalist propaganda may have left them largely untouched or unconvinced. These women did not think of themselves as "baby machines," or as machines of any sort, even when they least wanted the child that had just arrived. Pragmatic though they might be, so that offered the opportunity a good many might have elected abortion, they were not life-rejecting, and motherhood had its compensations even in the worst of circumstances.

Most of my ghetto informants, it seemed to me, were capable of both giving and receiving love in a way quite uncomplicated by ideology. For that generous capacity, sustained much of the time in difficult conditions, I salute them; and for the trust they placed in me, I deeply thank them. I can still see many of their faces in my mind's eye -- and no two of them are alike.

Barbara Frankel
Philadelphia, Pa.

TABLE OF CONTENTS

LIST OF TABLES

CHAPTER I

INTRODUCTION

The work upon which the present writing is based was originally and primarily intended as a fieldwork exercise for the development of certain indispensable skills in a fledgling anthropological investigator. Its fruits were meant to be more methodological than theoretical, and its orientation from the outset was inductive rather than deductive. I did not go into the field with a clear problem to solve, although, of course, I was aware that there were numerous problems which might be encountered, both of a methodological and theoretical nature.

Such problems were, of course, encountered, and were I to design the study over again there are certainly many things that I would have done differently. I cannot claim to have solved all the problems that arose in the course of the study and in drawing my conclusions, but merely to have made the effort and to have attempted to remain within the limits warranted by the nature of my data. Perhaps it is one of the more useful aspects of an exploratory study such as this one that it can indicate where the problems lie in the field under investigation, and thus lead to a more knowledgeable formulation of designs for future research.

The most central of the problems here is that of defining the unit of study. I have assumed from the outset that my informants, fifty American Negro women from the so-called ghetto area of North Philadelphia, represent a subculture with certain distinctive characteristics which remained to be discovered through investigation. Now, the definition of the term "subculture" is one of the knottier questions confronting anthropological theory at present. In particular, the designation of lower-class Negroes or other groups of the poor as constituting separate subcultures has been attacked theoretically as a distortion of the whole culture-concept, and politically as a means of blaming poverty on the poor. (Cf. Valentine, 1968:15) Nevertheless, even those who object to the "culture of poverty" concept originated by Oscar Lewis (1966) and who are most reluctant to attribute to all or even most poor people, white or black, the personal and social disorganization he describes do not deny that there are probably distinctive cultural adaptations which "animate the existence of those who live in poverty." (Valentine, op. cit.:16).

There is no intrinsic reason why the culture designs which characterize the poor--in this case some of the black poor of a large northern city--need be seen in pejorative terms. Indeed, it would be extremely strange if these patterns proved any less viable or adaptive for their bearers than those of any other segment of society. Whether poverty itself is deplorable and disadvantageous for those caught in it is not at issue. One hardly need state that the world would be a better place without it. But since the anthropologist, like any other scientist, must deal with what is rather than with what should be, the culture of those who inhabit the lowest stratum of our indubitably stratified society is certainly a fit subject for inquiry. It is viewed here not as something separate or immutable, but as something integral to American life as it stands today, and quite as mutable as any other aspect of a rapidly changing society.

Four major variables define the group of women with which I am dealing here. They are all poor, they are all socially defined as black by the larger society, they are all childbearing females, and they all inhabit a delimited geographic area which places them as urban dwellers. In a society structured as ours is, their race and poverty tend to act as isolating factors. Their urbanism, on the other hand, and the fact that they are females who share the function of childbearing with females of other races and classes tend to be factors which integrate them with members of the larger society. In the fact that there are means of daily contact and communication with the rest of American society, and in the fact that all mothers share certain basic orientations and common interests, this integrative tendency can be said to balance off against the isolation imposed by poverty and blackness.

The focus of the present study is on a single aspect of the culture of female ghetto dwellers, the folklore of the procreative process and infancy. It is my belief that the lore of a life crisis will prove fruitful as a means for arriving at valid generalizations about certain characteristic value orientations and core concerns of the ghetto subculture. The underlying hypothesis, of course, is that folklore--any body of folklore, but in this instance a specific genre traditionally called "superstitions" --can be analyzed as symbolic expression of such central orientations and concerns, and that therefore the lore has genuine significance for the student of culture.

Of course, if the lore of childbirth is to be analyzed as a culturally revealing phenomenon, it must be seen also as one which constantly grows and changes in response to changing conditions in the lives of those who transmit it. There will, therefore, be many items in the collection contained in the body of this thesis which will strike readers as odd inclusions under the rubric of "superstition" because they are obviously modern and scientific. For this reason I must make clear here that "superstition" refers not to a kind of belief (i.e., traditional as against modern) but to the general form of the beliefs--it is a generic term rather than a pejorative descriptive one in the present context. There will be further discussion of the genre problem, as well as of the problem of defining folklore, but for the present I merely wish to caution the reader to avoid thinking of all folklore as something left over from the dark ages, and to think of it instead as an emergent phenomenon showing the same dynamic aspects as any other part of culture.

Ruth Benedict, although she mistakenly conceived of folklore in static terms, and believed that "real" folklore was bound to die under the impact of modern civilization, nevertheless perceived with great accuracy the usefulness of such material to anthropologists. "Behavior and attitudes become more articulate in folklore than in any other cultural trait, and folklore tends to crystallize and perpetuate the forms of culture that it has made articulate," she wrote in 1937. (pp. 291) If this is true, as I believe it to be, the task of the anthropologist interested in folklore is not merely to collect, but to make inferences from his collection so that the values underlying "behavior and attitudes" may be laid bare, and the essence of culture itself therefore revealed.

Implicit in the statement above is a view of culture which sees it as a symbolic system which exists within human minds and is communicable at various levels through language and other communicative processes. This is the view which should be kept in mind throughout the reading of this effort: culture is composed, according to this view, of ideas at several levels of abstraction. At the highest level is what is often called the "world view"--the notions of what is real and unreal, meaningful or meaningless, true or false, knowable or unknowable in the phenomenological world around us. Somewhat lower on the ladder of abstraction, and limited by the nature of the world view at all times lie the values, the notions of "the ought"--of right and wrong, good and bad, pleasurable or painful, desirable or undesirable. Still further down on the scale lie what Kluckhohn (1958) called "cultural directives" and what most others call norms--the rule book full of specific sanctions for valued or dis-valued behavior which exists in every society, but is as often honored in the breach as in the observance, so that students of culture have had to distinguish carefully between these, the "jural" norms, and the statistical norms of daily behavior. It is the cultural, rather than the behavioral norms which will be considered here, in the main, though reference to the latter can hardly be avoided.

A word on methodology is in order here, before I proceed to detailed consideration of the data and the inferences which may be drawn from it. Cultural anthropologists have often been attacked by critics from other disciplines on grounds of design and sampling errors. The anthropologists have traditionally defended themselves by asserting that their interest lies in culture, not in statistical norms of behavior, and have said in effect that their aim was to choose an intelligent sample rather than a random one. (Cf. Mean, 1955) This defense has not always satisfied the critics, either within the discipline or outside it. (Cf. Wallace, 1961:89 and Mandelbaum, 1953:182) In the last decade or so, therefore, two trends seem to have developed in fieldwork methodology in answer to the shortcomings inherent in participant observation as traditionally employed by fieldworkers. One trend involves a degree of conversion to quantifying techniques. The other involves restriction of the field of inquiry sufficiently so that very precise and thorough presentation and analysis of data is possible, even in the face of that enormous complexity which characterizes cultural phenomena.

I have made some use of both approaches in the study undertaken here. I have, where possible, avoided statements of the order "most people say" and instead indicated how many people have said so, under what circumstances they have said it, and what the characteristics of these people are. Thus where general statements about values are made in the conclusion, the specific beliefs from which these statements are inferred are indicated, and the reader is free to look under the appropriate number to see which informants said it, and in the appendix to see what the characteristics of those informants were. In addition, by restricting the field of inquiry to a single aspect of culture, related to a single life-crisis in the female life cycle, gathered in a single setting, I have been enabled to present the data fully enough so that the basis for my interpretation of it might be wholly clear, and so that alternative interpretations might be possible. I believe that whatever validity may be claimed for my conclusions is an outgrowth of the care exercised in marshalling the data in such strictly limited terms as these.

One further purpose of the present study might be mentioned. Black Americans have, all too often, been viewed by social scientists merely as "victims of white prejudice. Blacks (are) almost never described in their own right as people or an ethnic group engaged in normal pursuits. They (are) described only as deviants." (Whitney Young, quoted by Leo, 1968) Since there is no situation more normal or universal than that of procreation, and since throughout this study I have sought never to lose sight of the great human significance of this event for each of my informants, perhaps it can be seen as a contribution which remedies to some extent the situation of which Mr. Young, quoted above, so rightly complained.

I should like to acknowledge with gratitude the tolerance and charity of my informants, who allowed me to transcend with them the boundaries of difference which set us apart from one another, and to enjoy the sense of our shared humanity and our shared motherhood. I should also like to acknowledge the generous help which I received throughout the course of the study and the preparation of this thesis from Drs. Jacob Gruber and John Szwed, who served as my thesis advisors. Thanks are due, too, to Dr. Russell R. De Alvarez, who allowed me to work in the ward, and to numerous members of the hospital staff who befriended me and made my work infinitely easier and more pleasant. To my husband and children, of course, who tolerated my preoccupied state over many long months, there is no adequate way to express gratitude.

CHAPTER II

THE SETTING

Temple University Hospital is a large, inner-city teaching hospital serving two health districts in North Philadelphia. The maternity patients I interviewed there come predominantly from an area bounded on the north by Erie Avenue, on the south by Spring Garden Street, and extending east to west from 3rd Street to 33rd Street. Only four of the fifty patients interviewed live outside this densely populated heart of North Philadelphia, and two of the four live only a few blocks beyond its fringes, in neighborhoods more recently "turned," but not essentially much different from the core area. Much of this area is slum in varying stages of decay, with a number of housing projects and a few blocks of "redevelopment housing" scattered through it. The great preponderance of North Philadelphia's inhabitants qualify as low-income families, if not as actually "poor" under the current Federal guidelines.

The hospital building in which the maternity ward is located is an elderly red brick structure five stories high. It is due for demolition in about four years, when a large new hospital complex will be erected in its place. Despite the imminence of its destruction the building has recently undergone extensive and much-needed renovations, and the old wards which once contained fifteen beds or more have been done away with.

When I first appeared on the scene the main OB ward was housed in the section called Four Main. This was a cheerful, newly renovated floor containing fourteen rooms of which four were private, one had three beds, one four, and the remainder had two beds apiece. All the rooms were individually air-conditioned and painted in soft colors. The nurses' desk was at one end, overlooking a glass window which gave onto the largest of the rooms, in which patients needing careful watching (but not isolation) were put when necessary. The private rooms were used for isolation cases or for overflow patients, and other patients were placed in whatever beds were available. At full capacity Four Main accommodated twenty-seven mothers with their babies, and all babies except those less than a day old and those in need of special care roomed in with the mothers. A conference room at the end of the hall was used to show films twice a week to educate mothers about birth control and infant care.

Four Main was the scene of forty of the fifty series of interviews which I conducted with informants between August 1968 and early February 1969. During this period, the delivery room was located in another part of the hospital, and I did not interview patients or observe in that domain.

The move to Three Main took place at the end of November. Some of the ward personnel, as well as patients who had earlier stayed on Four Main, experienced the move as a bit of a comedown at first, for Three Main possessed only one isolation room, and the six remaining rooms contained four beds apiece and lacked full height

MAP OF NORTH PHILADELPHIA AREA WITH LOCATIONS OF INFORMANTS' HOMES

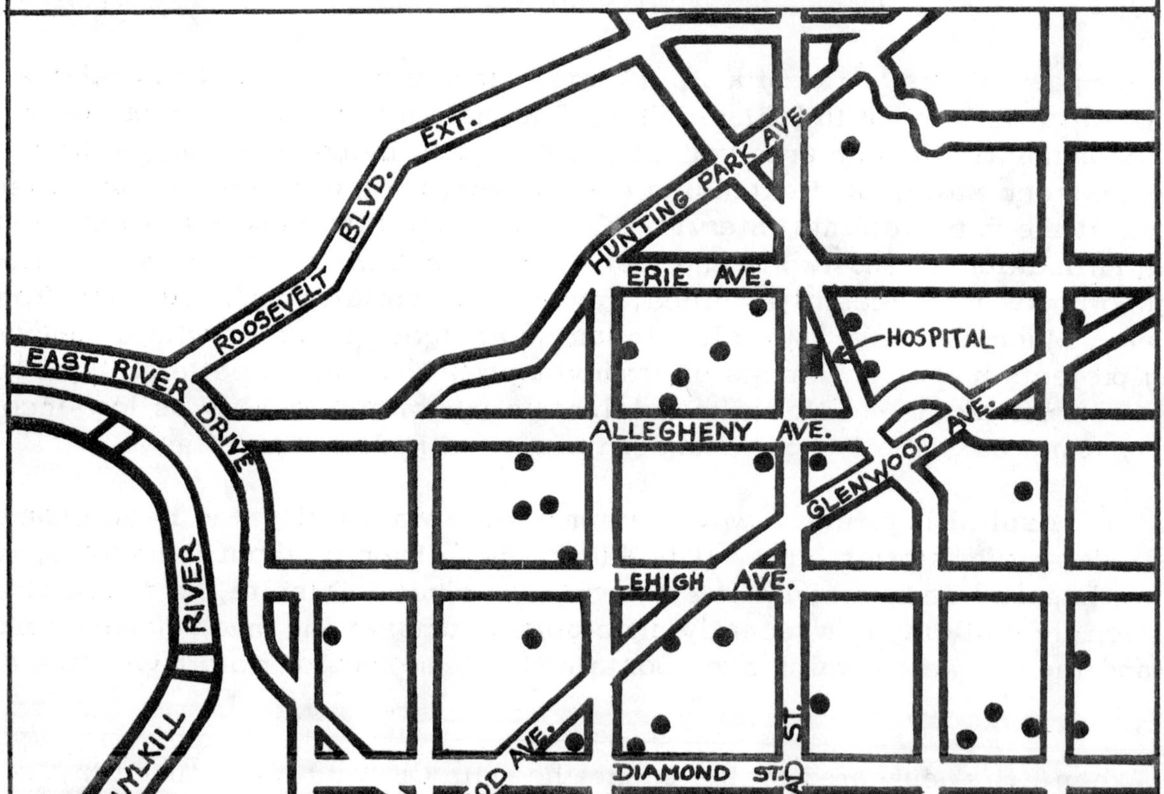

partitions between them. This led to a few complaints from "old patients" that the new ward was noisy, and less comfortable than Four Main had been. Nevertheless, Three Main would strike the average visitor as a cheerful, roomy, and pleasant place, even though its smaller conference room made the twice-weekly educational films rather cramped affairs if all the mothers attended.

During the daytime hours in which I usually visited there were two Registered Nurses, several practical nurses, and a number of nurses' aides on duty, as well as a ward clerk and two ward maids. In addition a procession of senior medical students, internes, residents, staff doctors, nursery personnel, supervisors, social workers, and records clerks from various departments were in and out all day long, supplying various services to the mothers and children. Food was hospital food--dull but edible--and special diets were given those patients who were in need of them. Staff members seemed sufficient in both numbers and training to give decent care to patients.

The attitude of most patients whom I was able to observe was undemanding in the extreme--in fact I can think of only one of my own informants who ever complained about anything not directly connected with physical symptoms in herself or her child to anyone in authority.[1]

The staff appeared to accept as a matter of course that patients should make few demands, and were, I thought, rather baffled by the occasional patient who didn't conform to this expectation. Still, on the occasions when they perceived some unreported distress in a patient there was a real effort made to offer help and support. On the other hand, hospital routine here, as elsewhere, didn't always allow staff members to become aware of a patient's distress, particularly if it wasn't strictly physical. Low-echelon personnel such as nurses' aides, or even maids, were likelier to be aware that a patient was worried or depressed than were nurses and doctors, for they were oftener in and out of rooms with a moment to chat, and were viewed more as equals by the patients. These people, however, seldom bothered their superiors by relaying information of this kind. Perhaps they shared with the patients a certain fatalistic acceptance of a degree of misery as unavoidable.

Typically, patients in the ward had attended prenatal clinic at TUH for anywhere from two to fourteen visits, usually beginning during the second trimester of pregnancy. About 85 per cent of the ward patients are Negro, reflecting the racial composition of the district served by the hospital, and almost all the rest are Puerto Rican. About 2,400 babies are born each year at TUH.[2] An estimated 95 per cent are fully or partially covered by some form of financial aid toward the costs of pre- and post-natal clinic care, prescriptions, and the usual five-day confinement.[3]

There are several forms of publicly-supported medical aid available to low-income women of the hospital district. They include three state and federally financed programs: DPA (Department of Public Assistance) coverage and Pennsycare, both of which involve some form of means test, and MIC (Maternal and Infant Care Project, administered by the City of Philadelphia) which does not involve such a test. The last named program can be applied for whether or not the patient has some other form of coverage, so long as she lives within the geographic district assigned to this hospital, and so long as she registers for clinic care before the end of the sixth month of pregnancy. There is, however, a limited monthly quota of patients who can be taken under the MIC program. Since certain benefits, such as homemaker services and birth control method of choice are available only to MIC recipients there are many assistance-wise women who apply for this program even though they are covered by some other program as well. Although a means test is not necessary for admission to the MIC program, there is a schedule of incomes beyond which the patient is not eligible for the 60 per cent of in-patient costs which are paid for the neediest families. (See income schedule in Appendix)[4]

The usual routine of hospital care for women whose pregnancies were uncomplicated consisted of monthly visits to clinic up to the last month or so, weekly visits thereafter until the time of delivery, a five-day confinement for childbirth and recovery, and a six-week postpartum checkup for both mother and child. Birth control information was routinely given during the hospital stay, and whatever method the mother might choose could either be taken home with her at the end of her confinement or obtained at the six-week checkup. Mothers who qualified for aid under the MIC program were entitled to receive birth control materials free for at least the first six months after birth of this child--after which they had to pay costs of such items themselves, unless they were DPA recipients entitled to free prescription services.

There is precedent for conducting anthropological investigations in institutional settings. (e.g., Henry, 1963; Goffman, 1961) Most of these, however, have been conducted for purposes of examining the culture of the institutions per se (e.g., homes for the aged, schools, mental hospitals) rather than the culture or cultures brought to the institution by its inmates, from the world outside. The present study is, therefore, somewhat of a departure from earlier studies done in institutions in that its aim was not primarily to examine the patterns of interaction within a hospital, but rather to use the hospital as a source of supply, as it were, for suitable informants, and as a relatively neutral territory in which to interview them.

Basically, the need to use a neutral territory such as the hospital was a function of my own position in the society relative to that of my informants. As a white, middle-class investigator I could "fit in" on a hospital ward in a way that would not have been possible in the homes of my informants where, indeed, my presence might have been resented as an embarrassment or worse.

Then, too, this was the normal setting for the particular event in the women's lives that I was interested in--having babies. Even the estimated 40 per cent of North Philadelphia's ward patients who do not register for clinic care seldom plan on actually giving birth at home. (Drake, 1969 interview with Dr. Batts of TUH) In the inner city of this day and age, women seek hospital care for childbirth. Home deliveries are rare and usually accidental, and even where these do occur the mother and child are usually taken to the hospital immediately following birth.[5]

Another advantage of the hospital setting lay in the fact that I was not occupying time which would otherwise have been economically useful to the informants. On the ward women were not busy keeping house, cooking meals or caring for older children. Time, in fact, hung heavy on most patients' hands, for there were no amusements and nothing to do. Women were expected to stick close to their own rooms, however, in order to care for their babies, and it was against the rules to carry them about to other rooms. My visits, therefore, were usually viewed as a welcome diversion.

There were, of course, some disadvantages inherent in the situation as well. The setting was emotionally neutral and appropriate to the event, but it was also unavoidably institutional, and I had reason to suspect that some of my informants, especially the young girls who had never before spent time in a hospital, felt rather ill at ease in this surrounding, and were therefore perhaps less spontaneous in their expression than they might otherwise have been. It was, furthermore, not the home the informants were used to--and since homes can be very revealing in a number of ways, I regretted my inability to make home visits in all but one case.

Since the average length of a hospital stay was only five days, and follow-up visits at home were not the rule, the use of this setting precluded the establishment of long-term relationships with most of the women who served as my informants. Nevertheless there was, in this atmosphere, a kind of "shipboard" quality to all relationships which led to a sometimes startling degree of intensity and confidence. This, however, is perhaps better discussed under another heading, later on.

FOOTNOTES--CHAPTER II

[1]On three occasions which I can remember this nondemanding attitude was directly responsible for new mothers becoming quite depressed when, due to an oversight on the part of someone in the nursery, their babies were not shown to them immediately after birth. All three convinced themselves that there must be something wrong with the baby, even though they had been told that all was perfectly normal. All three were afraid to mention that they hadn't yet seen the baby, and to ask that it be brought in. When I intervened and made the request it was willingly complied with. In one such instance, however, a patient commented that she believed this had something to do with my being the person who asked.

[2]Estimates provided by Dr. R. R. De Alvarez, in private interview.

[3]Estimate provided by Dr. Shulman, in private interview.

[4]All of my informants qualified for in-patient benefits if they were MIC cases. Thus the upper limit of incomes for these patients is within the scheduled limits for the program, so far as can be determined.

[5]This statement must be qualified to exclude the undetermined number of women and girls of whom I often heard tales--possibly apocryphal in some cases--who give birth at home, then discard their infants in a sewer or trashcan. One informant who lived in Raymond Rosen Homes, a large, high-rise apartment project, maintained that bodies of newborn babies were regularly found in the incinerators there. One such, she said, had recently been found alive by a janitor who was about to set fire to the trash, and police later located the fourteen-year-old mother, who had not yet borne the afterbirth. "The only reason the baby wasn't dead," said my informant, "is she came down to the first floor instead of dropping it from the twelfth, and it landed on a pile of papers . . . Nobody even knew she was pregnant, not even her own mother, because she was small and she wore girdles the whole time, so nobody noticed."

CHAPTER III

THE INFORMANTS

In all, fifty-nine persons were actually interviewed in the course of my research, but the group selected as fitting the design which I finally settled on for the study numbered just fifty. All fifty of these women were American Negroes, all were mothers or expectant mothers, all belonged to what may be classified as a low-income group, all had given birth to their babies in the hospital (and all but two were registered at clinic as well), and all resided within the area euphemistically known as the inner city. In other respects, they were as variable as any other group of urban dwellers. They varied as to age, religion, birthplace, length of urban residence, marital status, number of previous children, degree of social dependency, education, and such imponderables as personality and intelligence.[1]

My informants did not constitute a "group" in the sense that they knew one another before the time of their hospitalization, or had any sort of ongoing relationship. They are referred to here as a "group" for lack of a better word for referring to them collectively--perhaps Schneider's "bunch" of informants would be a more appropriate term. (1968:8) There was, therefore, no real social structure into which my informants fitted at the time during which I was able to observe them, save that provided by the hospital structure and routine, which brought a fleeting set of patient interrelationships into being--usually confined to the inhabitants of a single room, but sometimes extended to two or three adjacent rooms.[2]

Population Represented

The total number of people living as family units of which my informants are representative turned out to be equal in size to many of the villages reported upon in traditional ethnologies. My fifty women came from households in which 298 persons were reportedly living at the time of the study. (There may have been a few more, but almost certainly not fewer than this number.)

Of these 298 individuals 163 were children being raised by my informants, mostly their own offspring, but a scattered few were someone else's children. There were also a number of other children in the households of informants, usually younger brothers and sisters being reared by the informant's mother, but since I have no data on their ages I have not counted them among the children. (For a detailed tabulation of the composition of the informants' households, see the Table of Informants in the Appendix.)

Degree of Urbanization

Taking the length of urban residence as a rough index, this group qualifies as a highly urbanized one. Two-thirds of my informants had been born and raised either in Philadelphia (28) or another major northern city (5) and had spent all their lives, therefore, in urban ghettoes. Fifteen of my informants had been born in the South, and all but two of these were rural in-migrants to Philadelphia. There was only one informant who had been in the city for only one year, and four whose residence was about two years in North Philadelphia. All the remaining informants not born in Northern cities had been here from four to nine years. Two came from small northern towns, and one listed no birthplace and didn't tell me how long she had been here.

Education

Half of my informants had been through eleven or twelve years of formal schooling, and three others had a year or two of education past high school. Another thirteen women had from seven to ten years of school. Nine of my informants avoided stating their educational background on their clinic registration forms, for reasons unknown to me. Of this last group I suspect that at least two may have been functional illiterates, but I have no reason to believe that the rest were very far from the norm in general educational level.

By and large, then, it seems fair to classify the group as a whole as at least technically literate. They are all able to read labels on supermarket shelves, function in a money economy, sign their names, and some gave evidence of real interest in information gained in the past from reading. I didn't count the cases, but many if not most of my informants bought newspapers and pulp magazines when the cart came round to the ward in the afternoons (and one woman rather shamefacedly bought comic books). Some showed interest in the "dream books" sold on newsstands in the ghetto, and others giggled over "dirty books" they passed around among themselves. Many possessed "name books" to help them name their babies.

It is probable that boredom led many women to do more reading in the hospital than they generally would do at home. My point, however, is that where the need and interest arose my informants were, in the main, capable of reading for information and for pleasure. This, of course, has an important bearing on the folklore concerned with childbirth, for it would indicate that the printed page may well be the original source for some of what is later transmitted orally.

Fecundity

Thirteen of my informants were in TUH to have their first baby. One had just given birth to twins, her eleventh and twelfth children. These constituted the extremes of parity for the group, and a chart follows which details the situation for the rest of the informants.

An examination of the parity chart on the next page reveals that, as one might

TABLE 1

PARITY OF INFORMANTS BY AGE

Number of Children	Ages 15-19	Ages 20-24	Ages 25-29	Ages 30-34	Ages 35-42
1	7	4	2	0	0
2	5	4	3	0	0
3	1	6	1	1	0
4	0	4	2	1	0
5	0	1	0	1	0
6	0	0	1	1	0
7	0	0	0	1	0
8	0	0	1	0	1
9	0	0	0	0	0
10	0	0	0	0	0
11	0	0	1	0	0
12	0	0	0	0	1
Total Number in Age Group	13	19	11	5	2
Average Number of Children	1.5	2.5	3.8	5.0	10.0

expect, most of the primiparous mothers belong to the youngest age group, with the consequence that the fifteen-to-nineteen year old mothers had an average of only 1-1/2 children apiece. In the twenty-to-twenty five year old group, in which the largest number of my informants fall, they average almost 2-1/2 children apiece. In the twenty-five-to-thirty age group, the average goes up to almost four. In the group ranging from thirty to thirty-four there is a sharp drop in the number of women, but they average five children each; and my two remaining older women have a whopping eight and twelve offspring, respectively.

Despite the fact, then, that two-thirds of my informants are under the age of twenty-five, with many fertile years ahead of them, they already have an average of more than three children apiece--a figure that seems high compared to other urban populations. (Cf. Statistical Abstracts for U. S., 1968).

Social Dependency

Although all of the women in my sample of the ward population fall into a low-income category, they are not all equally dependent on public aid for medical expenses connected with childbearing. Twenty-nine of them, or almost two-thirds, are DPA recipients--a status which can be assumed as being totally dependent. Sixteen were receiving MIC aid from the city under a classification entitling them to full benefits, i.e., their income fell below the cutoff point for in-patient benefits. (See MIC Income Limits in the Appendix) There was, as has been pointed out earlier, some overlap here with DPA recipients, some of whom wished or required benefits not provided by the state. Five had other financial resources, either through the program known as Pennsycare, through a husband's union benefits, or social security payments. The two last named cannot, actually, be thought of as dependent statuses, since they derive from funds into which the recipient and his employer have paid. Social Security payments to this age group, however, do not carry medical benefits with them, so these were perhaps the most hard-pressed of all my informants when it came to payment for medical care.

The remaining mothers in my group (6) had no coverage of any sort, and must be assumed as being independent of the usual sources of social assistance--that is operating outside the system in some way which I cannot determine from the data at hand. Two of these were unregistered at clinic, and were brought in as emergency cases already in labor. Such mothers are almost certainly among the poorest in the neighborhood, since they have managed without prenatal care entirely. The remaining four were, to judge from their sources of livelihood, certainly eligible for some sort of aid on a financial basis, but had somehow missed out through too-late registration at clinic or through ignorance of application procedures.[3]

In summary, then, it seems that fully 16 per cent (8) of my group of women are expected to pay for the costs of their prenatal care and confinements. This figure is considerably higher than the estimate given earlier (see p. 7) of the percentage of maternity cases at TUH which are uncovered. The reasons for this are not determinable with the data at hand. In the totally dependent category so far as medical costs are concerned fall all DPA and Pennsycare patients,--and these women constitute 62 per cent of my group. The remaining women have other kinds of full or partial coverage, or some other indication (such as social security as the primary source of family income) that they are, indeed, in very low income brackets.

Family Organization

A table showing the composition of the informants' households by type of head appears on the next page and from this it can be seen that ten of the households under discussion are headed by the informants, another six by the informant's mother or other older female, thirty are headed by a husband or other adult male living with the informant, and four are headed by the informant's father. Fifteen of my informants live in households in which three generations are present, though it may be the informant herself who is the head of such a household. Thirty-four of the households are headed by an adult male, although six of these are categorized by the informant as her "boyfriend" rather than her husband, and may possibly be peripheral rather than integral parts of the households. In the female-headed households, as would be expected, the teenage girls tend to live with their mothers, whereas informants who are past twenty have left their mothers' households and are in charge of their own. Most of the women in the latter category have been married at some time.

Comparison of figures like these with census figures for the white population, or even with those for the non-white population, indicates that the incidence of the so-called "matrifocal household" (under the Solien definition, Cf. Kunstadter, 1963) among my informants is extremely high: 32 per cent of my informants live in such households as against 9.1 per cent of the white population of the U. S. and 23.7 per cent of the non-white population. (U. S. Census Bureau. ; 968:36) It is possible to speculate that such families may, perhaps, be positively adaptive in the economically marginal group studied here.[4] In any case, despite the high rate of occurrence of such households, it is well to take note of the fact that they do not represent anything like a majority of my informants. There are still 68 per cent of my informants who live in households headed by an adult male, and all but four of the thirty-four male-headed families were headed by the husband or consort of the informant. Thus, a majority of my informants appear to be living in what would at least statistically appear to be standard American nuclear families, a few of them with older relatives included in the household.

Child Care Arrangements

Although recipients of MIC have homemaker services available to them during their confinements, none of my informants in this category took advantage of this--perhaps because they didn't know about it, and perhaps because they preferred to leave their children with relatives if possible. Of the thirty-seven women in my sample who had other children one did not have her older child living with her, and the other thirty-six had to make some provision for the care of other children in their absence. Twelve had their mothers looking after children, and four their mothers-in-law. Five women had left their other children with a sister, and eight more had an assortment of other females, both relatives and non-relatives, doing the babysitting. In only three homes was an adult male left in charge: one an elderly, retired husband, one a crippled brother who lives with the informant, and one a young husband who took his vacation in order to babysit.

In most of the cases where the children were left in the care of a person who

TABLE 2

COMPOSITION OF INFORMANTS' HOUSEHOLDS
BY AGE GROUPS AND TYPE OF HEAD

Age	Informant	Older Female	Husband or Consort	Older Male
15 - 19	1	6	3	3
20 - 24	4	0	14	1
25 - 29	3	0	8	0
30 - 34	1	0	4	0
35 - 42	1	0	1	0
Total	10	6	30	4

Female-Headed Households:	16
Male-Headed Households:	34
	50

was not a regular member of the informant's household, the children were taken to the home of the babysitter for the duration of their mother's confinement. (See Table of Informants in the Appendix) Several of the mothers expressed uneasiness about the competence of the person who had been left in charge--particularly when this was a male, or a younger female family mother. It was evident that, probably in common with most other mothers in the U. S., informants preferred to have an older female family member as a babysitter in their absence, ideally a woman who had raised children of her own, but was no longer the mother of many young children herself.

Religion

Religious distinctions among my informants were not great, and seemed to have little bearing on their responses during interviews. Two declared that they had no religion, most were Baptists for the official records, and there was a sprinkling of other Protestant denominations and of Catholics. Only in the case of the last-named group did their appear to be any modification of views which might be connected with sectarian religious belief, and this was, as might be expected, expressed most directly with reference to birth control. It must, however, be pointed out that negativistic lore on this subject was by no means confined to my Catholic informants, although they were most liable to express moral uneasiness in specific terms.

Generally speaking, I have the impression that my informants live in a highly secularized moral universe, at least one in which denomination mattered little. There was no particular item or type of belief which appeared to set off one religious group from another. This is not to say that elements of religious feeling are not present in the beliefs--for they are, indeed, in the strong feeling about the sacredness of motherhood and its obligations, in the reliance on a higher power in times of stress, and so on. Nevertheless it seems fair to say that an early speculation of mine about the possible determining role of a woman's religious upbringing in forming her attitudes and beliefs about the reproductive process was not borne out by the data.

To summarize the character of this group is not easy, for it would seem to be more notable for its variability than for its uniformity. Nevertheless perhaps a few general statements can be made with safety, beyond those which were made at the outset concerning the group's fixed parameters of race, residence, motherhood, hospitalization, and low income.

This is a group which is generally rather young and reproducing at a rate which is well above the level necessary to maintain the population. The preponderance of its members are thoroughly urbanized and rather secular in outlook. They may be classified as literate, also, though the degree of literacy is variable. Although there are indications of rather low stability for marriages in this group, marriage is still the norm, and most informants have been married at some time. Families still tend to be headed by men, even though a very sizeable number are not. Naturally enough, since this is a very low income group, there is a high degree of social dependency, with over half my informants in the totally dependent DPA category. It may be superfluous to note that there is nothing particularly suprising in any of this--numerous studies of the American Negro poor attest that most of the characteristics of my group of informants can be found among similar groups elsewhere, and studies of the urban poor of many corners of the globe present a picture which differs in only a few details (e.g., literacy and the availability of social services, which are less widespread in non-western countries).

On the impressionistic level, I cannot overstress the wide range of types my women represented in my contacts with them. There were the cheerful and the depressed, the passive and the aggressive, the malicious and the kindly, the gallant and the defeated, the contented and the miserable, the suspicious and the friendly--in short, even though all my informants were more or less in the same sociological boat, they navigated that boat in very different ways and with very varying success.

FOOTNOTES--CHAPTER III

[1]I refer here to personality and intelligence as "imponderables" because I made no attempt at measuring these factors by means of projective tests, I. Q. tests, or other measuring instruments. Such an attempt, I felt, would not only be unduly time-consuming but also would change the nature of my relationship to the informants in a way that might interfere with the pursuit of my major objectives. I did not wish to appear in the role of a "testgiver," to whom "right" or "wrong" answers might be given.

[2]Only once did I hear of any active "social" relationship developing on the ward. This occurred when several patients who had spent extra days in the hospital for various reasons, managed to send out for beer and threw a party for themselves one night which lasted into the small hours of the morning. A lively time was had by all, and telephone calls were made and received by the participants until well past midnight--which caused some complaints from patients who weren't involved, and a good bit of stir among staff members the next day.

[3]The Social Service Department of the Hospital makes every effort to keep the latter category of cases at a minimum, in the interests of both the patient and the hospital, but a few always slip through. In cases where the patient is too late registering, or misses being included in the MIC quota and is not quite destitute enough for state aid, she is referred to the business office to work out a plan for payment. In the past, of course, many such bills were in default, and I am told that the hospital now employs a collection agency to keep after them.

[4]Newman, in fact, maintains that matrifocality was the preferred family structure among many of her Negro clinic patient informants in California (1965:192-194) Szwed (1969:unpublished) suggests that the lower class Negro in the New World may, in fact, be characterized by a type of adaptation to low status and economic deprivation which entails individual networks rather than solidary family groupings.

CHAPTER IV

SELECTION AND INTERVIEWING OF INFORMANTS

My procedure for obtaining information was rather simple and straightforward. On interviewing days I spent anywhere from six to eight hours in the hospital, about half this time being devoted to the actual interviewing of informants, and the rest to consulting records prior to initial contact with them, and to recording the data immediately after our conversations.

Before going into any patients' rooms for the first time I consulted their records at the nurses' desk, and briefly noted those identifying features and vital statistics which I felt I would need. These always included the patient's name and address, room number, age, birthplace, religion, marital status, data on the child's father and the patient's previous children if any, relevant details of the new infant's birth and condition, number of prenatal clinic visits the patient had made, kind of aid or other plan for payment to the hospital, and the date the patient was due for discharge.

The sampling of patients was basically random within the parameters already described earlier for defining my group. I did not attempt to "design" my sample in order to make it a perfect cross-section of the female inhabitants of the locale from which the informants were drawn, nor even of the OB ward population, which was not exclusively Negro, as has been mentioned earlier, nor even exclusively very low income. My underlying assumptions were that the twin factors of blackness and poverty did, in effect, act as boundaries for ethnic identity among my women, and that this particular ethnic group has a distinctive subculture. Other than these, the only selection factor was sufficient time for at least two interviews before the date of a patient's discharge.

Interviewing was done in patients' rooms, since they were expected to remain there most of the time in order to care for their babies. There was no means of insuring privacy in rooms where there were two or more patients, other than by drawing the curtains around each bed--and the privacy which this would have assured was merely visual. I had reservations about the utility of creating such a bogus "privacy" for my interviews, for not only would it have been no real privacy at all, but I felt that it would unduly dramatize my presence and create rather than eliminate barriers to the kind of rapport I wished to establish. I did not, therefore, attempt to interview my informants singly by design, but instead encouraged small group sessions which included all the patients who happened to be in a room at the time I walked in. This necessity turned out, in the end, to be a virtue, for the atmosphere created by the informants themselves was usually that of a relaxed "hen-party" in which everyone swapped their experiences and knowledge about the interesting business of pregnancy and childbirth.[1]

Usually there were two to four women present during interviews. (The larger groups were more characteristic of the latter part of my study, when the new quarters on Three Main made four beds per room the standard number.) Occasionally, despite the fact that the staff frowned on too much circulating of patients between rooms, women from elsewhere on the floor dropped by and joined in the festivities, so that there were sometimes as many as five or six persons present. Such sessions became exceedingly animated, as shy patients were drawn in by the bolder ones, and women competed with one another to demonstrate their knowledgeability in the arcane matters of female procreation and infant care. Thus I found that the context was more natural and the sessions more productive when I followed a rule of "the more the merrier."

Two assumptions lay behind my strategy in approaching my informants. First, that since these women were both poor and black they might very well harbor a certain resentment and suspicion toward white, middle-class authority figures. Such attitudes could conceivably have wrecked the whole project, so I had to exercise some care in winning the women's confidence. I could do very little about being white and middle-class. I could, however, do my best to present myself in as non-authoritative a light as possible.

In the interests of so doing, I made a point of avoiding being seen by patients in conversation with such upper-echelon staff members as doctors, nurses, or social workers, although I frequently consorted with maids and nurses' aides, who sometimes joined briefly in our "hen-sessions." I also made a point of presenting myself as a student rather than as an august professional. This was not only the truth, it also left the matter of my precise status open to interpretation. Since graduate students were an all but unknown breed to the ward patients, they usually simply assumed that I was working toward an undergraduate degree. Also in line with this approach, I decided early in the course of my research to eliminate note-taking during interview sessions, on the supposition that this might identify me in the informants' minds with teachers, DPA visitors, or even policemen--all of whom are authority figures who are prone to write things down.

My second assumption is really a corollary of the first. This was that in their contacts with authority figures from the middle-class white world many of my informants had probably suffered ego-bruising experiences--had been made to feel ignorant, stupid and inadequate on many occasions. If this assumption were correct, I must win trust and establish rapport on a premise that would be ego-building rather than the reverse--an application of the old saw that you can catch more flies with honey than with vinegar. I therefore explained my study to the women in such a way that they were cast in the role of my allies and teachers--as indeed was the case.

The formula I used went approximately like this:

> I'm being let into the ward here to talk to all the mothers I can, because to tell you the truth, I'm trying to settle a friendly argument with some doctors I know. You see, I have an idea that women who are mothers know a lot more about having babies than most doctors give them credit for--after all, women were having babies for thousands of years before there <u>were</u> any such things as doctors or hospitals, and somehow the human

race managed to survive. So what I'm trying to do is find out as much as I can about what all the women here actually know about having babies--how they get started, how to take care of yourself while you're pregnant, how to get through the labor, how to take care of the new baby--all you can think of that's connected with childbearing.

Having thus established sexual solidarity at the expense of the medical profession and of men in general, and having also let my informants know that I believed they really knew things that would be both of value and of interest to me, the interviews usually proceeded in lively fashion from there. Quite regularly the little speech paraphrased above brought forth vigorous assenting nods and smiles along with remarks like: "That's right! Women know things about having babies that no man in this world can know anything about."

Interviews were informal and open-ended, with no rigid schedule of questions employed. I had, however, a general outline of topics in mind throughout the interviewing stage, and managed to cover these pretty well with all but a few relatively uncommunicative informants. It was both logical and convenient to arrange my general topics chronologically, opening with a question such as "When you were small, what did your mother tell you about where babies come from?" From that starting point it was simple to progress to what they later learned to believe when they were past the age of "stork stories," and on to the other topics. The four major areas of inquiry covered can be summarized as follows:

1. Conception: how it takes place, how one knows that it has taken place, how one might go about preventing conception or inducing it, and factors which are thought to influence fertility or sterility in women.

2. Pregnancy: including information on its normal course, possible abnormalities of pregnancy, hazards to the welfare of mother and/or child, means of insuring the welfare of mother and child, means of terminating unwanted pregnancies, and prenatal influences on the unborn child.

3. Parturition: including beliefs concerning what may constitute normal or abnormal courses of labor, influences which may ease labor or make it more difficult, the legitimate role (magical or otherwise) of persons assisting at childbirth, and the role of mother, father and child in the birth process.

4. Postpartum: including beliefs about proper care during the confinement and in the early weeks at home for both mother and child, means of dealing with illnesses or other problems during the early postpartum stage, and customary patterns of reliance on others (friends, family, social agencies) during this time.

As I have mentioned earlier, I did not take notes during interviews because I wished to appear non-threatening and to allow for the most relaxed atmosphere possible. For the same reasons I didn't employ tape recorders or other recording equipment--which I did experiment with on one occasion and found to be inhibiting to my informants. This remark is not intended as criticism of those who have, often very successfully, employed recording devices in ethnographic field work--and certainly such equipment would greatly have simplified my task in many ways. The use of such devices, however, has generally been confined to two types of situations: those where the chief focus was on verbatim collection of fairly long and complex genres of folklore, and those where the investigator had first been able to establish fairly long-term relationships with the informants as a resident in their community. (Cf. Abrahams, 1962 and Eddington, 1968, as well as numerous others.)

In my own situation, however, I was interested in a very simple and easily-memorable genre as it could be elicited in as relaxed and natural a setting as I could create. Furthermore, my period of acquaintance with all but a few of my informants was confined to their five-day stay in the hospital--not long enough for most people to overcome their inhibitions in the presence of recording devices in the hands of a total stranger.

There is ample precedent for refraining from direct recording of interviews and other events in ethnographic literature. Usually such a strategy is chosen where the informants are literate and know or sense the implications of the written word for social control exercised over them by persons of superior status. Mean (1932) employed this kind of field methodology in her study of the "Antler Tribe," although she expressed reservations about it in a later introduction to that work. Powdermaker, in Stranger and Friend (1966) also describes use of this technique in her work among Mississippi Negroes, and Diaz (1966) followed a similar procedure when she worked at Tonala. There have been many others, no doubt.

As all of the investigators mentioned above have pointed out, the content of a conversation, if it is not too prolonged, can be memorized well enough for a quite good transcript to be made of it if such a transcript is done immediately afterward. Diaz comments that she found herself, if events lasted longer than an hour or so, threatened with "imminent mnemonic confusion." (1966:10) My own tolerance in the field situation was a shade better, and I found that I could do a good job of recording conversations lasting up to an hour and a half. Perhaps the reason for my own greater time leeway lay in the fact that I was not recording events which were perfectly free-wheeling and naturally occurring, as she often did at Tonala. All of my interviews were, of course, different from each other--but they all covered much of the same ground, and there was also a high degree of redundancy in the folk beliefs themselves. In addition, I never had to deal with really large numbers of people at any single session--nothing, for example, comparable to recording a complicated ceremonial involving dozens or even hundreds of people, or a party where everyone might be talking at once.

At least two interviews were conducted with each informant, and each of these lasted anywhere from an hour to an hour and a half. In some cases I found a particular informant especially interesting in terms of her knowledge of the lore of childbirth, and made it a point to spend more time with her than with other informants who were less productive. The two-interview stipulation, then, is merely a lower limit, not an upper one.[2]

Initially I planned on two interviews per informant with the idea that the first session would be merely a "warmup" in which I would establish friendly relations and get some notion of the patient's personality and interests, leaving the major data-collecting for the second meeting. Actually, however, I found that the two interviews were not very different in the quantity of folklore they produced. The novelty of the whole undertaking operated from the start, almost, to produce a spate of information from most of the women--especially those who felt that they were rather authoritative when it came to having babies and raising them. A day or so of thought following the initial conversation, however, seemed to allow many women--even those who had at first been rather shy--to recall things which hadn't occurred to them earlier. It seemed, then, that the first interview served to skim off the most common and widely current beliefs and prescriptions, while the second served to plumb a deeper level of memory and to deal with matters that were more arcane and unusual. The latter often included things the women refused to believe or were rather frightened of because they half-believed them. I think, too, that the very fact of my returning a second time encouraged trust and the feeling that I was <u>interested,</u> which also operated to stimulate people.

Of course, as soon as I felt myself threatened with the mnemonic confusion of which Diaz speaks, I made as quick an exit as I could manage, and headed straight for my office corner and portable typewriter. There I worked madly for as long as it took to make as complete a transcript as possible of the contents of the conversation --separately for each informant--the interplay between participants being indicated by the use of codes for cross reference, and my own reactions and impressions being added at the end and designated as such. I also took care to record the behavior, insofar as I was able to observe and note it, that accompanied various items of conversation: the smiles, groans, shrugs that may change the entire meaning of a statement.

There are, of course, certain disadvantages to having so brief a relationship with an informant as I had with most of mine, and I cannot claim to have mined the depths of the individual personalities--or of the culture--of my informants under the conditions I have described. Nevertheless I must call attention to a phenomenon which I sensed, though I cannot prove, as inherent in the circumstances of the sort of research I was doing. For lack of a better word I call this the "shipboard" quality of the relationships which are established when a group of total strangers find themselves thrust together in a common situation. Here, sharing a significant life experience with people one will probably never see again, many of the defenses people conventionally need to employ can be temporarily discarded, and a remarkable intensity can sometimes develop in relationships between very disparate kinds of people. It is to this factor that I attribute the sometimes-remarkable confidences to which I was made privy, for I would hesitate to attribute such phenomena to any special skill of my own and am otherwise at a loss to explain the utter trust which was sometimes placed in me.

Female ethnographers have generally been in an advantageous position, of course, for the collection of the female lore of any society, for reasons too obvious to bear repeating. Even in our own society, where male doctors generally do minister to the needs of parturient females, it is still rather easier for women to discuss childbearing and child-rearing among other women than in the presence of men. Much of the data presented here would not, I believe, have been available to a male investigator--and the fact that I was not only female, but also a mother like themselves, gave my informants and myself a real universe of common experience which was perhaps the most valuable research tool of any that I possessed.

FOOTNOTES--CHAPTER IV

[1]If, as Ben Amos maintains, folklore itself should be defined as a process of small-group communication (1967:19) the fortuitous use of a small-group context may have been more than helpful. It may, indeed, have been essential to provide a situation suitable for the "folkloring" process itself. (See section on Approach, p. 27)

[2]The upper limit, in truth, would figure to an astronomical number of woman-hours, for like most anthropological field workers I had my one "special favorite" informant. This was an exceptionally bright and articulate woman who also happened to be a severe diabetic, and who therefore spent many weeks at a time in the hospital throughout her pregnancy and afterward. My relationship with her has been a very close one on more levels than the professional, and I am deeply indebted to her for many insights into ghetto life.

CHAPTER V

AN ANTHROPOLOGICAL APPROACH TO "SUPERSTITION"

Professional scholars of folklore have traditionally published their collections with heavy annotations and cross-references to the collections done by their fellows, largely in the interests of tracing the origins and diffusionist careers of the items they have collected. This mode of scholarship reveals, of course, the heavily antiquarian bias of folklore scholarship which dominated the field until rather recently.[1] Only in the last decade or so have younger scholars departed somewhat from this tradition and focussed upon context as much as upon text--but they too have tended to perpetuate the pedantries of historical scholarship, even where these were hardly relevant to their central concerns.[2]

I should like to state at the outset that my concern here is not with the histories, conjectural or actual, of the beliefs which I have collected, however interesting. As an anthropologist doing a non-comparative study, my interest is focussed on the way in which the beliefs function in the lives of my informants at the present moment, and with the way in which this functioning may illuminate their culture and perhaps culture generally. I am, therefore, not concerned with whether or not a belief is traditional. Many of them are as new as yesterday's newspaper containing the latest article on birth control, though many are quite obviously much older. What is traditional is the <u>process</u> for communication of beliefs, and the form or <u>structure</u> through which they are communicated. In the broadest sense, the <u>function of beliefs</u> such as these probably remains the same through time, in that they satisfy needs for understanding and at least partially controlling events of a crucial nature. (Functions of specific beliefs may, of course, shift over time as their credibility wanes, and they may come to have more value as entertainment or as sentimental ties to the past than as genuine "lore," or knowledge.) <u>Content</u>, on the other hand, may and does alter in adaptation to the state of society and of the knowledge available to the "folk"--and in this sense folk beliefs may be thought of as a continuously emerging phenomenon, rather than as collections of quaint antiquities.

There has been an enormous amount of scholarly disputation over the years as to what is and what is not folklore. The dispute has led to some absurdities of inclusion and exclusion which are ably reviewed by Ben Amos and need not be dwelt upon here. In the end he resolves the dilemmas posed by "the definition game" by suggesting that folklore be defined not as a <u>thing</u>, but as a <u>process</u>--a communicative process, to be precise. This process, he maintains, is distinguished from other sorts of communication by its artistic form and by its typical occurrence in small-group or "reference group" contexts. Thus, "folklore is the artistic communication in small groups"--a definition broad enough to include non-verbal forms (such as music and dance) or even written forms (such as "slam books" and graffiti) as well as the present genre. (Ben Amos, 1967:19)

Ben Amos has surely set things on the right track in introducing the notion of process into the definition of folklore. I would, however, lean toward qualifying the use of the term "artistic"--both because I am not certain that there are or can be any cross-culturally valid canons of art, and also because it would be difficult to call the present corpus "artistic" by any canons whatsoever--though I would stoutly defend it as being folklore. I would, then, amend Ben Amos's definition by changing the word "artistic" to "stereotyped" or perhaps "non-casual" as Abrahams (1964:92) and Voegelin (1960) have used the latter term.[3] In essence, however, I find the definition proposed by Ben Amos to be the most operationally useful of many encountered, and with the emendation noted above, it is the one to be kept in mind here. "Folklore," then, "is the stereotyped, non-casual communication in small groups."

To sum up, I consider that the present corpus, though evidence of the process just discussed, also exhibits three other aspects which may be conceptualized as distinct, and which indeed are implicit also in the definition. Discrete items display structure (implicit in their non-casual nature), function (implicit in their use within a given context, the small group) and content (implicit in their being defined as a form of communication.) The first three aspects of the lore (process, structure, and to a lesser degree function) may be thought of as "traditional." The last, content, need not be--it can easily be the new wine which is poured into old bottles. These four aspects are, of course, always inseparable empirically, but it is helpful to view them as conceptually distinguishable.

Most of the classic collections of folklore represent a tradition of scholarship which, honorable though it is, differs importantly from the current anthropological tradition and its concerns. Such collections have, therefore, usually been made under conditions very different from those of the present study. In the older collecting tradition, with few exceptions, only minimal attention was paid to context, while major attention was devoted to the absolute authenticity of the verbal record. This has meant that tales, riddles, superstitions--or whatever--have had to be elicited in such a manner and under such conditions that they could be recorded word for word. The verbatim standard has, in fact, become so much a part of unquestioned dogma for all kinds of folkloristic researches that recorded texts (before the advent of really modern tape recorders, which have to a degree freed scholars from certain handicaps of an earlier age) have usually not been taken from the spontaneous expressions of the informants in a natural setting, but more often have been written down or recorded under highly artificial conditions after the collector's first hearing of them, by appointment, in a quiet place, and generally alone.[4]

There may be ample justification for this procedure where the collector's chief interest is in the literary rather than the cultural values of folklore, and where the idiosyncratic "folk artist" is therefore more interesting than the "average" group member. This sort of isolation of the folkloric event from its context is, however, of very dubious value to anthropologists, whose interest is culture--and to whom, therefore, it is not only the text but the occasion and the group which are important.

Since the focus of this study is not art but culture, and since, for reasons explained earlier, I did not think it advisable to employ either notes or tap recorders during interviews with the patients at TUH, I cannot lay any claim to having collected here precise verbatim transcriptions of the folk beliefs of my informants. I can and do, however, lay claim to essential accuracy and to having done the collecting in that natural, reference-group context which Ben Amos (1967:19) has suggested, quite rightly I think, as one of the defining criteria for the communicative process which is inseparable from the meaning of folklore.

I do not consider that the partial scuttling of the verbatim standard is, in this instance, a serious handicap. For one thing, this particular genre, along with such genres as riddles and proverbs, is by its simple structure and brevity quite easily memorized for as long as it takes to make a good transcript afterward. The memorability of so-called superstitions is, in fact, one of their signal characteristics. For another thing, although this genre of folklore has quite a precise implicit structure, this structure is often explicitly violated in the actual telling. Thus the same belief may be forthcoming in several forms with no confusion at all as to the fact that the belief is always the same one.

An example of this phenomenon would be, perhaps, a belief whose "generalized" form may run like this: "When you are pregnant you skin gets lighter." One informant may, however, tell the collector "My mother says you can tell if somebody's pregnant, because your skin gets lighter." Or, perhaps in answer to the collector's question "How do you know when a woman is pregnant?" the informant might say "They says your skin gets light, or something like that." Or, again, an informant may launch into a longish tale of the way in which she tried for several months to conceal the fact that she was pregnant, only to suffer the chagrin of having a friend or relative tell her "I knew it all along--your skin got lighter."

Newman points out that the validation of belief through personal testimony is "a venerable tradition in Negro folklore."[5] (1965:131) The form of such beliefs is what Honko calls a "memorate" (1968:11); that is, a first- or second-hand tale which acts to rationalize and actualize some belief held by the informant. A great many of the beliefs presented here were first given to me in the memorate form--indeed perhaps a majority of them were. It would, however, be impossible within the limits of this report to transcribe verbatim all the tales within which the beliefs were encapsulated. Such an undertaking would, indeed, have required recording equipment to do full justice to the material--as well as several hundred pages added to this thesis. Where the memorate is very brief (as, for example, where informants begin a succinct statement of belief with "My aunt knew I was pregnant before I did, because . . .") I have included it in full. Where, however, the belief is found within a long and complex tale I have merely summarized it following the identifying number of the informant and the letter indicating my estimate of the level of her belief. (See Pp. 65-66 for discussion of levels of belief.)

I would suggest that some strategy such as this one has been employed by most collectors in this genre.[6] The reasons for so doing are obvious. The verbatim publication of five or six minor variations on the same single-sentence "superstition" would be both tedious for the reader and taxing for the scholar. It would, indeed, be mere pedantry--since it would not serve any really useful purpose for either literary or scholarly researches. A superstition is not, by and large, ordered in a manner that can be termed "artistic," either by its users or by anyone else--it doesn't build to any climax, or satisfy any particular aesthetic. A full-scale "memorate" may, indeed, be a tale of some complexity--but since the focus here is on the beliefs and not on the story-telling skills of any particular informant, the consideration of these has been left to one side for present purposes.

By and large one finds that so-called "superstitions" constitute a simple, pragmatic kind of category. They are established on the base of cognitive needs, for we cannot act unless we know. These beliefs, then, are means of dealing with life events, not means of heightening or embroidering upon them. Even those which sound most occult to modern, educated ears are, essentially, no more nor less than the lore (or knowledge) of the folk (or ordinary people of a society). The precise wording is seldom of weighty literary or cultural importance, although fidelity to the general style and spirit of natural utterance is, of course, desirable.

In short, I would take issue here with that brand of scholarship which might maintain that impeccable recording of possibly-unnatural utterances obtained under rigged conditions is preferable to less perfect recording of spontaneous utterances obtained in as natural a situation as possible. I have, therefore, chosen the latter course as the preferable one for anthropological purposes.

FOOTNOTES--CHAPTER V

[1]Along the lines of this tradition, see Puckett (1926), Botkin (1945), Brown (1952-64, but collected much earlier), Dorson (1956), and Browne (1958).

[2]In the newer mode one finds, most notably, Abrahams (1962 and 1964) and Goldstein (1964a & b), as well as Ben Amos among folklorists. Anthropologists interested in folklore have, of course, often taken a synchronic approach--although Herskovits (1941) and others were interested in the survival of lore over great spans of time and space.

[3]Voegelin, however, maintains that training is required for the production of the utterances he would term "non-casual." In the present case, the use of the term "training" would surely be an overstatement of the process through which the lore is learned. I would, however, maintain that the lore of childbirth is learned through a process which might be termed "initiation" over a period of time beginning with or shortly before a woman's first pregnancy, and extending into the early months or years of the childrearing phase.

[4]Such a course of action on the part of the collector is, indeed, specifically enjoined by Y. L. Cahan (see Bauman, 1962) as well as other mentors of students of folklore. See also Goldstein's 1964 manual for collectors of folklore, where this technique is also suggested, even though considerable thought and emphasis are given to collecting in context as well. Dorson (1956) too, describes such out-of-context collecting in detail and with some pride in his scholarly rigor. Boas, among anthropologists, employed similar techniques, as did Ruth Benedict and other Boas students. This may account for the relative neglect of their material by later anthropologists as, somehow, intrinsically useless.

[5]Dr. John Szwed has suggested that this may, in fact, be true of all folklore traditions, not only that of American Negroes. As a form of knowledge, it seems only natural that people would attach to it various proofs of truth and efficacy.

[6]Dundes, for example, in "Brown County Superstitions" (1961) attributes any number of the listed items to more than one informant, and one to no less than four different individuals. My own experience with informants would indicate that, in fact, it is very rare for the same belief to be couched in precisely the same words by two different informants, even when they are together during the interview. Usually one will paraphrase the other rather than repeat her words exactly. I must, therefore, assume either that Dundes' experience differed radically from mine, or that he has done what Goldstein calls "generalizing the belief into its 'proper' form"--a practice which he warns against. (1964a:15)

Since Dundes has not been explicit about his methodology, however, one is left wondering whether, indeed, the beliefs are in a generalized or synthesized version of what he was told by informants, or whether he has, alternatively, simply chosen the "best" version from among several versions of a single superstition which were given to him. In other words, there is no way to determine from his remarks whether any actual human being ever spoke the words he has ascribed to one or more persons. Dundes is by no means alone in having done this, of course.

The difficulties which this situation has raised for me lead me to be more explicit than most collectors have seen fit to be regarding the form in which the belief finally appears here. In order to avoid cumbersome repetitions of essentially identical beliefs couched in differing vocabularies. I have selected the version of each item which is most succinct, explicit and complete, as nearly verbatim as I was able to record it. The first code number following the belief will be that of the informant whose words I am quoting, and other informants listed will be those who have given a phrasing which agrees precisely in substance with hers. Summaries of significant memorates accompanying each informant's presentation of a given item will be placed after her code number. Wherever there is any doubt as to whether a belief is, indeed, identical with another, they will be listed separately.

CHAPTER VI

PRESENTATION OF DATA

Some sort of classification system is, of course, essential to an orderly and comprehensible presentation of any corpus of data. It should also, ideally, be of such a nature as to facilitate analysis and assist in the drawing of conclusions.

Dundes has proposed one such system for this genre, which is conventionally termed "superstitions."[1] (1961) His is a threefold division based upon his definition of the genre in terms of grammatical structure as "traditional expressions of one or more conditions and one or more results with some of the conditions signs and the other causes." (Ibid.:28) This definition gives rise to three categories of superstitions: (1) Sign, in which the condition is a sign and the result an inevitable sequel to it, with man placed in a passive role; (2) Magic, in which the structural formula (if A, then B) is the same, but where the condition is created (whether volitionally or not) by human agency; and (3) Conversion, actually a sub-category of magic, in that it contains beliefs in which man has the ability to circumvent the outcome of signs or magic through some prescribed act.

Dundes' categories are suggestive, but perhaps less useful than would appear to be the case at first glance. It is, for example, difficult under this system to separate a sign (such as a natural event) from magic (such as an involuntary action by a human being). Indeed, it is not a structural distinction that must be made in such instances, but purely one of content. An example of this might be the attempt to draw a distinction between "If you're born in the wintertime you'll be coldnatured" (presumably a "sign" in Dundes' system) and "If you're evil when you're pregnant, the baby will be evil, too," (which--though involuntary perhaps--would come under "magic" because the agent is human and active).

A closer examination of this supposedly structural system, then, actually reveals that it is by no means based upon an independent concept of structure, but is bound up with both function and content at every turn.[2] I have, therefore, been forced to the expedient of constructing a system of my own which both fits my data better and makes assumptions which are simpler and more straightforward.

Mine is a basically functional classification consisting also of three major categories (plus one residual one containing material which does not fit into the three functional categories). The assumption which underlies this kind of classification is really a psychological one. This is that human beings in a life-crisis situation such as childbirth tend to feel a realistic anxiety, and that there are three major ways in which to reduce such anxiety: specifically through attempts at recognition, explanation, and control of the events taking place. In the present instance, culture supplies the means of anxiety reduction in true Malinowskian fashion, through folklore.

Recognition, of course, is basic to any further action--one must know what is happening before one can decide how to meet it. Thus, if the signs point to possible pregnancy, one must prepare for the event (or perhaps attempt to forestall it) through seeking out an expert such as a doctor whose specialty lies in this area. If the signs say that the baby will be a girl, one might buy a pink layette--but one must first know the signs so that one may recognize what has already happened, or predict what is going to happen. Following Dundes' usage, I have called this the category of "signs," although I have used the term somewhat more broadly to include anything which may enable one to discern or predict an event connected with procreation. Some signs are physiological, some emotional or behavioral, and others external to the individual--but all perform the same function of providing knowledge. Thus one may know that one is pregnant because the menses have ceased, or because one's disposition is suddenly "evil," or because one's grandmother has dreamt of fish--but all are signs of the impending event.

The second category refers to that tendency which not only Levi-Strauss, but many others note among all human groups--albeit in very different manners in different cultures--which leads men to seek causal explanations of the events which befall them. It may as yet be uncertain what are the bedrock "needs" which may define man's psychic unity.[3] Nevertheless, I found, among my informants, at a purely empirical level, a lively and pervasive interest in knowing not only what was going to happen, but why things happen as well. I have called the category of beliefs which display this central notion of causality, simply enough, "causes."

My third major category is in some respects rather similar to Dundes' category of "conversions," in that it has to do with the active response to some sign or cause. Since it is a functional category, however, I have chosen to call it the category of "controls" which one may, through right knowledge and action, exercise over one's present or future fate. Typically this pigeonhole contains beliefs which entail a remedy or prescription following upon recognition of a condition otherwise liable to cause grief. An example might be the statement of a teenager that if a boy and a girl "do something" together, the girl should protect herself against pregnancy with "something you buys at the drugstore." A "control" belief thus serves the function of conferring some degree of autonomy upon the individual, so that he is not entirely at the mercy of external (or internal) events.

There are, of course, always some difficulties with systems for the classification of essentially untidy cultural data. There are, for instance, minor problems in separating signs from causes. An example is the belief which says that a mother who suffers from heartburn during pregnancy will give birth to a baby with lots of hair. Sometimes informants state this in the form of a sign ("If you has a lot of gas when you're pregnant that's a sign the baby will have lots of hair") and sometimes as a cause ("Yes, he sure do have lots of hair--and he give me a-plenty of heartburn, too!"). In such cases as this, the belief will be listed under both headings.

There is also the matter of drawing distinctions between causes and controls. If, for example, one may cause a baby to be born ugly because one has laughed at an ugly person while pregnant, there is an implicit control present also. One need not laugh at an ugly person. The knottiest problems in this area are raised by matters of contraception: here the very essence of the beliefs seems to be connected with control--in fact precisely with birth control. Yet it is most common for women who have neglected to exercise this control to see their neglect as a cause for pregnancy--a view which is quite correct, after all. ("If you forgets to take the Pills--even for a day or two--you can end up pregnant.") In such cases as this, I shall allocate the belief to the category which seems indicated by the form in which it was given, and the evident meaning intended by the speaker.

Within the three major categories the beliefs and superstitions will be divided, for convenience in analysis, into content categories. Under signs, for example, will be ranged together all the signs of pregnancy, the signs for predicting sex, the signs that delivery is imminent and so on. This is done simply because the ranging together of like or contrasting beliefs on the same subject makes inferences about values and symbols which are important to the informants easier to make.

Cultural data being what it is, I must make mention of a fourth and final category--really a non-category--which contains a small store of comments, ficts,[4] notions which fit into no functional category, and direct value statements of a stereotypic nature that may help to illuminate the present inquiry a bit further. It is included because, despite the lack of obvious functional significance, there are elements of belief here which should not be overlooked, as well as indices to the likely behavior of my informants in particular situations (such as that presented by a child's questions).

Cultural inferences are not always easy to make no matter how material is organized--but as Goldstein tells us (1964a) it is not possible to make them at all unless we have some notion of the level at which a given belief is held by each informant from whom it was collected. To this end he has suggested a system of indicating the actual degree to which a superstition is believed. It is admittedly rough-and-ready, but will serve until more refined techniques are invented in the rosy future of cultural investigations. There are four levels of belief distinguished in Goldstein's suggested system for the collection of superstitious beliefs which I employ here.

(1) Total belief (though not necessarily one which is always practiced, I find) in which the truth of the statement is not doubted. This will be designated by the letter "T" following the informant's code number (s) after each item.

(2) Partial acceptance, in which there is some rejection of the belief at the rational level (perhaps influenced by the observer's presence, or fear of ridicule) but in practice the belief is not abandoned. For this level I will employ the letter "P."

(3) Humorous incredulity, in which the belief is intellectually rejected, but is nevertheless passed on to others for "fun." This, which is really a level of non-belief, will be designated "H."

(4) Rejection so total that the belief will not be normally passed on by the informant to others, and is usually expressed only because the investigator has elicited it by asking for items thought to be false. This level will be designated "R." (Goldstein, 1964a:17-19)

Informants, of course, will be listed (by code number to protect their anonymity) after each item of the collection. They are specified more fully in the Table of Informants in the Appendix, which gives a number of significant facts about their social status, education, and family situation for easy reference.

INDEX TO THE BELIEFS

I. SIGNS

II. CAUSES

III. CONTROLS

I. SIGNS

A. Signs of Pregnancy

In this category beliefs range from the most "natural" or medically verifiable signs to the most "occult" ones, such as prophetic dreams. All informants know, by the time they have been examined at clinic and told they are pregnant at least, that cessation of the menses is an early sign. A few, of course, reported putting other interpretations--hopeful ones, one must presume--on the fact that they had "skipped" once or twice. One informant, confused and ignorant at age thirteen, had managed in her youth to twist the facts entirely, and told me: "The first time I had a monthly I thought I was pregnant, even though I hadn't had nothing to do with no boys. I was scared to tell my mother. I was afraid she'd beat me, 'cause of thinkin' I was pregnant." (Informant 46, now the mother of eleven)

Between the purely natural and the distinctly occult beliefs lie many signs which shade rather gradually from one extreme to the other. Some of these, such as condition of skin, hair, and nails probably refer to signs of hormonal change which are actually observable in some individuals. Others may refer to fairly common symptoms of pregnancy such as anemia (6), nausea and swelling (4), or even rapid pulse (7), and the irritability which goes with toxemia of pregnancy or simply with fatigue (9, 10). It is in this middle ground of verifiability and universality of symptoms that, quite naturally, the levels of belief among informants vary most. It is here that women will almost always use testimonials to validate the truth of their belief--and to prove that they are not superstitious, but are willing to believe their eyes or someone else's, if only conditionally.

1. If you stop having your period, that's the first sign that you're pregnant. (1 T, 26 T, 35 T, 30 T, and 14 T who, however, says that her case was atypical in that menses continued for several months, making diagnosis difficult. 46 T reported that her sister refused at first to believe the sign because a doctor had once said she's never conceive. "So she just thought she was skipping a period, on account of she wasn't never too regular, you know." Informant 3, on the other hand, reported "The <u>first</u> sign I was pregnant--before I even missed my period--was when I started to feel sick to my stomach." Informant 16 declared, however, "I missed my period a few times, but I didn't know I was pregnant. I thought I had taken cold or something. When you take cold it can make you miss your period.")

2. When a woman is pregnant, her skin will clear up. (26 T)

3. When you're pregnant, your nails will grow faster than usual. (26 T)

4. If you're pregnant you know it because, even before you miss your period, your breasts get bigger, and you might feel sick, or either very hungry, or faint or something. (II. 3T reports similar signs, with the addition of cramps. Many women, of course, report such symptoms, but only these two phrased them as "signs.")

5. I knew by the third week I was pregnant. I knew because my gums would start to

hurtin'. They would get swollen like they never was any other time, and my whole mouth would hurt. They say lots of women gets the toothache, but I got real good teeth, so my gums started hurtin' instead. (36T)

6. When you're pregnant, they say your skin gets lighter, or something like that . . . (49P, 37T, 39T, whose mother told her this. Possibly this is objectively true--many of the ward patients suffer chronic anemia which is probably intensified by pregnancy and may, indeed, cause them to look paler than usual.)

7. My father knew I was pregnant before I even knew. He could tell by the vein in my neck. He said he could see a double heartbeat in my neck and that was a sign I was pregnant. (5T. Her roommate, informant 8, had heard, too, that "older people can tell when a girl is pregnant by looking at her throat" but wasn't sure she believed this.)

8. When a woman's eyes look real clear, and shinier than usual, that's a sign she's pregnant. (24P, who only half believes that her grandmother really knew in this way "before I knew it myself." Also 39T.)

9. When they's pregnant, some women gets evil. (41T, who adds, however, "With me it was my husband that got evil. I got real sensitive, and if my husband said a single word to me, I'd start to cry.")

10. When you're pregnant you want to get even with people. (36T)

11. When a young person is pregnant they will fade away from an older person (i.e., begin to act cool, even though they had been close previously). (5T reports that this is how her friend's grandmother knew she was pregnant.)

12. Now, my aunt always knows I'm pregnant before I shows or anything. She says it's because the only time I ever comes to visit her is when I'm pregnant--and that's true, too. I never do visit my aunt except right after I gets pregnant--sometimes before I know it myself. (49P)

13. When I was about eight I noticed my mother getting fat--the dress she always wore, one of them kind that wraps around and ties in front, started stickin' out in front and getting skimpy behind. My girlfriend told me that my mom was expecting, then, so I knew where the baby grew. (46T)

14. Some people can tell when you're pregnant by havin' a dream. (26T, who says that her "mother-in-law"--actually the mother of her "common-law husband"--had such a dream, but she didn't know its content.)

15. If you dream of fish, that means someone in the family is pregnant. (13P, 18P, 24H, 30T. Two informants phrase this as "someone close to you" rather than restricting it to family members.)

16. If you dream of a person going naked in front of people, that's a sign they're pregnant. (24T. This informant says that two of her girlfriends had such dreams

about her, even before she knew she was pregnant, within two nights of one another.)

B. Signs of Sex and Multiple Births

Although Newman (1965:135) found in her study of Negro and white private and clinic maternity patients that the Negroes and whites were differentiated from one another in the greater number of beliefs concerning means of predicting of sex among whites, my data contradict that observation. My group of Philadelphia Negro women offered a wide range of such beliefs, some of which I had never heard among whites, others of which appear to belong to a common corpus of lore which may well have world-wide distribution.[5]

Beliefs regarding sex prediction fall in the realm of the unverifiable. Few women say they really have total faith in these signs, yet despite only partial or merely humorous acceptance of them almost all were accompanied by testimony of some kind in the form of a memorate. This may be accounted for by the fact that for most of the signs there is an opposite form which is equally well known--therefore a mother may easily rationalize after the fact by recalling the signs she experienced, and taking these to be proof that she "knew all the time the baby would be a boy (or a girl)."

Women were about equally divided between those who preferred having girls and those who wanted boys, i.e., there was no statistical bias as to sexual preference. There was, however, outspoken preference for one or the other on the part of almost every mother. The typical middle-class "I don't care what it is as long as it's healthy" was notably absent. Furthermore, the reasons for a particular preference were highly stereotyped, and phrased in terms of informants' notions of what was good or bad about the respective sexes (Cf. Conclusion, pp. 102-4) even though sexual preferences were always phrased in terms of how much "trouble" a boy or a girl might be to rear.

Twins, of course, are actually predictable by means of X Rays and even through careful use of stethescopes. No one, however, mentioned either of these techniques of prediction. The only physiological means mentioned had to do with the size, in pregnancy, of the mother's belly. Other beliefs regarding twin births were really concerned with the manner of determining their sex. There was surprisingly little anxiety over the thought of having twins--in fact several women thought they'd be fun to bring up, and said they wouldn't mind having them, even though they are obviously "more trouble" than a single birth.

17. The doctors thought I might have twins, because I was so large this time. (14P, who did, however, have a single birth.)

18. If you carry high you'll have a boy, and if you carry low it'll be a girl. (1P, 18P, 24P, 26P.)

19. If you carries low it'll be a boy. (32P, who carried low, and had a boy.)

20. I knew it was going to be a girl because I carried high and round. (4T)

21. If you carry high and pointy it'll be a boy. If you carry low and round it'll be a girl. (31P)

22. I thought it was goin' to be a girl because I carried high, and everybody told me that's what it would be. (46P, who wanted a boy, but had a girl.)

23. My sister carried a girl high and the boy low--but I've heard it the other way around, too. (28H)

24. If you're going to have a girl you'll carry high and pointy in front. A boy gets carried low and round. (15T)

25. If you carries behind it'll be a boy, in front it'll be a girl. (31H)

26. They say if it lies on the right side the baby is a girl. (29P, 33T)

27. My husband's aunt knew I'd have a boy again this time. The baby laid on my right side and kicked a whole lot. (33T)

28. The old folks in Mississippi say that you can tell if you're having a girl or a boy by which side the baby is lying on when you're carrying it--but I don't remember which side is which. (20H)

29. I didn't know it was going to be twins. I sort of thought it was going to be a girl, but sometimes I'd feel the head up here on my right side, and sometimes I'd think it was over here on the left. I guess that was because they was two of them tangled together with hands and legs all over the place, so I really couldn't tell which side the baby was lying on. (39P)

30. You can tell if you're going to have a boy because a boy moves around more when you're carrying him. (7T, 42R, 32T)

31. They say that boys is lazy and don't kick so much. (36P, who had her third girl, declared "and this one kept kickin' me the whole time!")

32. A little part that starts to show in the back of your hair and won't go away is a sign the baby will be a boy. (18P)

33. If your hair falls out all during the time you're pregnant, the baby's going to be a girl. If your hair grows long and full it'll be a boy. (2H, 18P, 24H, 26P)

34. I knew it was going to be a boy because I felt good this time. (48T, who added that she felt good with all her boys, but "with my girl I suffered the whole time." Informant 46T expressed the same thought in almost identical words, saying "the girl gave me a lot of trouble--I had that false labor, you know.")

35. If you act evil when you're pregnant that's a sign the baby will be a boy. (27P)

36. If you is always acting evil when you're pregnant, that's a sign the baby is a

girl. (25T)

37. If you have a child at home that clings to you when you're pregnant, the baby will be the opposite sex from that child. (30T)

38. My friend's little sister didn't like her the whole time she was pregnant--that's how we knew she was going to have a girl. She was jealous 'cause another little girl was coming. (35T)

39. A girlfriend of mine had a baby girl, and when I picked that baby up it started in crying and wouldn't stop till I gave her back to her mother. That was another sign I was carrying a boy. (31T)

40. When two children cling to you while you're pregnant, you'll have twins--and if it's a boy and a girl, the children will be a boy and a girl, too. (30T)

41. My grandmother knew from a dream that I'd have twins, a boy and a girl. (30T, who also dreamed of twins--which is what she had--but in her dream both were boys. She believes in her grandmother's prophecies, rather than her own, because she is certain her grandmother is gifted in this direction, having predicted the sexes of all her grand- and great-grandchildren.)

42. I knew it would be a boy this time. I dreamt it would be a boy--in fact I dreamt of twin boys, though I'm glad it was only one. But I got the sex right. (14P)

43. I wanted a girl, but I kept dreaming, while I was pregnant, about baby boys. (31T, who believes in the prophetic power of dreams, had a boy.)

C. Signs of Imminent Delivery

The emphasis in this group of beliefs is less on specific "signs" than on feelings--whether vague or strong in nature--which many women refer to but cannot describe except to say "it's like an instinct . . ." or "I just had a feeling." When women get that "feeling" they frequently decide to get their houses in order against the time of confinement, and put in a strenuous day of washing, cooking, and ironing. Since this may in itself have something to do with hurrying things along at a very late stage of pregnancy, we have a self-fulfilling prophecy in all likelihood.

During labor a great many women express certainty that they know better than the doctor when the baby is actually going to be born--and not a few feel resentment that the doctors sometimes ask them to "hold back" to prevent precipitate delivery (and presumably tearing) or to allow time for a spinal anaesthetic to be administered. One woman said very forcefully ". . . and you can tell them doctors one thing. A woman knows when her baby's coming, and she can't hold it back, neither. They ought to listen when she tells them it's coming . . . Why, they ain't no way to hold yourself back when that time comes, and that baby wants to get itself born!"

44. When your naval drops you is ready to deliver any time. When that happens you

gets heavier down below and lighter up above, so you can eat your food without feeling full after a few mouthfuls. (20T)

45. A baby will be born the night the moon changes. (26T, whose labor began, she says, right after the full moon.)

46. You watch for the signs of the moon. A baby will always be born either at the half, or at the full, or at the wastin' away moon. (20P, who says her father, a half-Indian from Mississippi, "told me how to follow the old Indian custom to tell when my babies is due.")

47. I was sure scared that first time . . . The funniest thing that happened, though, was when I heard my pelvis open, after they gave me the spinal. I just heard a loud crack, like somebody's bones cracking, and soon the baby was here! (46T, who has eleven children, and has listened for this each time but has never heard it after the first delivery. Her conclusion: "I guess that only happens with the first one.")

48. When I dreamed of the delivery room every day for a week, I knew I was going to deliver, even though my time wasn't supposed to be for another month yet. (17T)

D. Signs of Inborn Traits or Marks

Most beliefs concerned with the baby's appearance or inborn personality characteristics are phrased as "causes" rather than signs and are discussed further under that heading. A few, however, do fit here.

49. If you have heartburn a lot when you're pregnant, that means the baby will have a whole lot of hair. (35P, 25T, 27P, 36H, 50T)

50. A person born with a veil (caul) will be able to see things. (15P, who told rousing "ghost" stories about her own family, but seemed not the least frightened by them herself, and indeed professed to be curious about but not afraid of the supernatural. I am not sure whether she should have been designated as "T"--her stories about her Aunt Eunice, a poltergeist, were mightily convincing.)

51. When babies is born with holes in their ears, they see things, but only while they are little. (42T, who claims to have a brother like this, was genuinely disturbed by the fact that her new baby girl had such a "hole," which turned out to be a tiny indentation, like a pinhole, just where the top of the ear joins the head. She says that her brother often saw things that nobody else could see before he was of school age, and once nearly fell out a top-floor window because he saw a dog outside "just in the air" and wanted to play with it.)

E. Signs of Fitness for Childbearing

Bearing children is, in this group as in innumerable other groups of women throughout the world, the supreme validation of femininity. By no means all, but many of my informants looked upon having a baby as their real coming-of-age (not, as is almost universal in the middle class, getting married). I am told that the term "virgin," among many of the teenagers of the ghetto, has come to mean not a girl who has never had intercourse, but a girl who has not yet borne a child.[6] If true, and if having a child also marks a girl's real entrance into adult status, these facts may in part explain the high rate of early (and usually illegitimate) pregnancy among ghetto teenagers, and also provides a clue to a very real and positive split between the mores of ghetto teenagers and those of the larger society. It would also indicate that some such early "mistakes" are sometimes not mistakes at all, and cannot be looked upon as such by the agencies charged with dealing with very young girls who are pregnant. Some of these pregnancies are, rather, an aspect of conformity to peer group standards among older adolescents. (Cf. Abrahams, 1964 comment on women's view of childbearing)

With motherhood valued so strongly, it is a matter of real anxiety if a woman is unable to bear children or shows signs of not being able to have as many as she may want. One woman, whose daughter was interviewed (she was having her first child at fifteen) had herself had twelve live births and several abortions. When, at thirty-four, she gave birth to twins, a tubal ligation was performed in the interests of her health. She found it necessary to tell people, though, including her own daughter, that she really hadn't <u>had</u> to undergo the operation. "She was as good as she ever was, and could have gone on having babies, only she didn't want any more."

52. People who miscarry just don't have a strong a system as some other people. (41T, who says "I quit work right away, as soon as I knew I was pregnant, after them two miscarriages I had.")

53. If you feels bad after the baby's born, it means you aren't too strong (for childbearing). (2T)

F. Signs of the Infant's Fate, or of Supernatural Intervention

It is not easy to separate some of these beliefs from items about inborn traits of an occult variety (such as 50 and 51). There is, however, a difference between someone who is gifted (or cursed) with some special "power" and simple "signs" that angels--or devils--may play with newborn infants sometimes. There is a widespread notion, seldom expressed explicitly but underlying many of the beliefs in this category, that babies are closer to heaven or hell than older people, and that their souls are less firmly attached to their bodies.[7]

This is a category containing mostly apparent "survivals" of an earlier time and an older belief system, without doubt, but there is beginning to be introduced here, too, newer lore based on statements from medical practitioners, as well. The first belief listed in this category illustrates this. It is interesting to note that in this instance the belief serves the function of comforting the mother for the loss of a child through emphasizing the hope every mother has that her child will be normal. (Most abnormalities, of course, appear under "causes.")

54. When you has a miscarriage real early, like I did, the doctors tells you the baby probably would've been born retarded, or crippled, or something like that. (42P, who nevertheless was most careful to avoid miscarriage, after two miscarriages, when she found that she was again pregnant. Interestingly, she had a baby who had six fingers on each hand, but ignored the deformity completely in the course of her conversations with me and with other patients. The defect was remediable, and she had been told this--nevertheless I was curious as to whether this represented an unusually easy acceptance of imperfection in her child, or whether it meant that she was blocking the fact that he was deformed. I was unable to get a clue--she seemed proud as punch, and seemed to think he was just beautiful, as indeed he was, otherwise.)

55. If the baby doesn't crawl before it walks, it'll crawl before it dies. (31P)

56. Dreams can tell you what will happen to the baby. (26T)

57. When my oldest son cried in his sleep they told me it was a sign the devil was chasing after him. (31P, who therefore used to pick the baby up to "chase the devil," just in case it might be true. Also 30P)

58. When the baby smiles in its sleep, the angels are playing with it. (30P, 31P, 42T, who thought it was a sign that the baby's soul was "too close to heaven, so that it might die, or something." She, therefore, made a point of watching over her baby very carefully at night, picking it up when it smiled, and also when it cried.)

59. If a premature baby is born in an odd-numbered month it will live, but if it's born in an even-numbered month it will die. (7R, 9R. Both informants denied this was true, and the first talked contemptuously of "all that stuff about lucky and unlucky numbers. Odd numbers is supposed to be lucky, and even one unlucky. But I knows the longer that baby is in there, the better chance it's got.")

60. A seven-month baby is supposed to live, and an eight-month one is supposed to die. (9R, who added "but I don't believe all that junk!")

II. CAUSES

A. Causes of Pregnancy

This category divides into two sub-sections: those beliefs which center around the physiology of sex, *per se*, and those which center on methods of birth control, their side effects and the failures of them which may result in pregancy.

The first category usually appeared in answer to the general, impersonally couched question, "How does a girl become pregnant, do you believe?" The second category, on the other hand, was elicited in response to the somewhat different question, "How did you get pregnant?" or perhaps "Do you know how you got pregnant this time?" The first question is, of course, more abstract, and can be answered without reference to any personal experience of the informant's. The second kind of question, by contrast, was usually interpreted to mean "How did you get caught?" and was usually answered in those terms, with some reference to a failure to use contraception properly, or a failure of the method itself. (I recall only one woman who said that she had thought it "time to give my husband another baby to bounce on his knee," and had therefore deliberately stopped using contraceptive measures, so that she would conceive.) Since mention of birth control methods usually elicited further comments on such things as side effects and efficacy I have also included these beliefs among the second sub-category.

It was not until I analyzed my data that I became aware of how crucial the phrasing of this particular question really was. The first, relatively impersonal question, didn't require an informant to discuss her personal sex life in supplying an answer. The second, on the other hand, could not be answered without such intimate discussion except by reference to contraceptive failure. In this situation, the informants generally chose to speak of a "slipup" in prevention of pregnancy, rather than refer directly to their own intimate behavior.

Sterility is not an area of primary concern for most of the women--not surprising, of course, since by definition these women are fertile. That their own fertility is important to them has been mentioned earlier in connection with fitness for childbearing. It is interesting, however, that a few women in the group interviewed, even though their major problem was fertility more than sterility, referred to the "fault" for sterility sometimes lying with one's mate rather than with oneself. The two mentions of a possibility of willful behavior leading to sterility were connected to the general disapproval and fear of abortion.

Birth control information is now generally available to women who attend TUH clinics or are confined there for delivery, and an active program of birth control education is carried on in the ward, as had been mentioned earlier. This has, I am told, been in progress for about two years. One must assume, therefore, that the knowledge of contraception abroad among the ward population is rather recent in origin. This fact makes it doubly interesting and revealing that my group of informants possessed such a mass of information about the subject. The mothers in the ward, generally speaking, know much more about the whole range of birth control methods than I would expect an equivalent-size group of middle-class women to know. The educational films and lectures which almost all ward patients attend during their confinements (if only because they are bored, and this passes for entertainment) are explicit, accurate, and give a full range of necessary information on this subject. Few middle-class women are treated to this sort of educational program. It is paradoxically likely, therefore, that this group--so long denied access to means of regulating family size--is now more knowledgeable on the subject than is much of the middle class.

Of course, any subject so vitally interesting as contraception would be in the lives of poor women becomes the subject of much word-of-mouth transmission of information, as well. This accounts for all the knowledge, and the many testimonials, concerning side-effects of various methods and their relative efficaciousness. Some of this information may be garbled, but much of it is also quite accurate, and acts to help people in making intelligent choices for their own use. On the other hand, the many "scare stories" about side-effects sometimes operate to make women fear to use any method whatever--even though they know a great deal about contraception in the abstract. Older women, particularly those whose early pregnancies date from the time before general availability of this knowledge, are usually the most conservative in this respect. They would often "rather bear those ills they have than fly to others that they know not of." It is usually the older woman with numerous children--(in a bit of picturesque medical parlance called a "grandmultipara")--who at last resorts to tubal ligation to bring an end to her numerous pregnancies.

1. Conception and Sterility

61. If a man and a woman have sexual relationship, that's how a woman gets pregnant. (8T, 31T [who told the story below in belief #71] and 46T. In fact, this knowledge is universal, virtually, by the time a woman is in the hospital for confinement.)

62. If a man and a woman sleeps together, the woman can get pregnant. (34H, who chose to take the term literally, then laughingly added "of course, if all they're doing together is sleeping, ain't nobody going to have no baby!")

63. I told each of my (older two) daughters when they first got their monthlies, "Now you can have a baby, so don't play with no boys." (46T, who wasn't sure this was the right tack, because one daughter's response was laughter, and "Is that right?")

64. If you pleasures yourself with a man, you'll get pregnant. (20R, who added sadly "That's what they told me down home in Mississippi--but I done been pregnant eight times, and I know I didn't have no pleasure every one of them eight times when I conceived.")

65. You can get pregnant from just one little drop (of semen.) (11T)

66. If a girl who isn't pregnant laughs at one who is, she'll soon be pregnant herself. (26P, who says, "and that's what happened to me, this time! I laughed at my girlfriend, and a month later, there I was.")

67. If nature takes it course, you're likely to have a baby every year. (36T, who adds "and that's just too much!" Her grandmother, who raised her after her mother died, disapproves of interfering with God's will by means of contraception, but this young woman has decided that she will have her babies when she wants them and can provide for them.)

68. When my mother's cousins adopted me and my brother, it must have brought them good luck--because they never had any children of their own before that, but they had a little girl about a year after they took us in. Adopted children brings good luck in the house, they say. (28P)

69. If you have the wrong mate you might not have any children. (13T, a widow who never became pregnant while married to her husband, nor with a first "boyfriend" whose five children she later adopted. She now has three of her own, however, by a second "boyfriend" who moved in when the first left.)

70. If you can't have a baby it ain't always the woman's fault. Sometimes it's the man. (9T)

71. Trying to get rid of a baby is dangerous. It might mess you up inside. (29T, 46T, who has a cousin who reputedly had several abortions in her youth and about whom she commented "I guess with all them abortions she done messed up her seed or something. I don't think she can have none now. Look like she'd be lonesome at her age without even one child.")

2. Contraception, and Its Side Effects and Failures

72. I was on the pill for two years, when I stopped taking them for one month because I had no money to buy them. That month I had sex, then I missed my period and I knew right away I was caught again. (31T, who discovered, too late, that she could have obtained a DPA prescription which would have been filled free of charge. 49T told a similar tale, in which similar events had been responsible for the birth of all three of her children, "but the last one took a whole year before I got pregnant, I don't know why." 46T stopped taking the pill because "it messed up my periods" until she began to have symptoms serious enough to warrant a D and C [curettage, a minor surgical procedure]. Following her operation but before resuming the use of the pill "I had intercourse, and I got pregnant right away--and here I am.")

73. This is a change of life baby. I was taking the pills. Then I missed my period twice and went to the doctor, and he told me I was probably starting in to change life and I should stop taking the pills. So a few months later I was pregnant. (32T)

74. If you forgets to take the pill even for a little while--like, say, a day or two--you can get pregnant. (18T, 11T, who spoke of "forgetting" too, but actually discontinued taking the pill because she suffered nausea, dizziness, and a weight gain of fifty pounds which she attributed to it.)

75. If you takes the pill <u>regular</u> you can't get caught. (24T, who added "but I didn't so maybe this time I'll get a coil instead.")

76. The pill can make you get all fat and sloppy-looking. It can make you sick to your stomach, too--or you can get dizzy spells from it. (11T, who preferred tubal ligation to other contraceptive means--an unusual choice for a woman of 24 with only three children. 36T added to the list of side effects that some people "gets nervous or has headaches. Some people even claim they can give you cancer." 35T gave testimony on behalf of her sister, who "had a whole lot of blood clots on her stomach, and she had three periods in one month and gained 45 pounds in six months." For this reason the informant chose to get an IUD. [Intrauterine device, often called "the coil."] 6P mentioned weight gain and blood clots. "I knew a girl that had one that travelled to her heart.")

77. I'm afraid to get a coil, because a coil might could hurt. (9P, 11T)

78. A coil can fall out without you knowing it, and then you can get pregnant. (7T, 9T)

79. After the coil is put in you might have some cramps for a while, like menstrual cramps, but these go away. The important thing to watch for with a coil is to make sure it doesn't fall out. (26T, who adds that in the latter event "you have to come back to the hospital to have it put back in, or you'll get pregnant." This, of course, is a "control.")

80. A coil might make you feel sick to your stomach. (11T)

81. Them older women, they think everything's going to cause you to get cancer. My mother told me I could go ahead and try it if I wanted to, but she wouldn't, because she'd heard a coil could give you cancer. (46P, who never did get around to getting an IUD, because she believed in being on the safe side, evidently.)

82. A coil could grow into the lining of the womb, and a woman would need an operation to get it out. (36T, who claims she knows a woman to whom this happened, and who developed all the symptoms of pregnancy due to the implantation of the IUD in the uterine wall.)

83. A coil might could cause an infection. (7T, 9T--both of whom gave this as their reason for not wanting to employ this method of contraception.)

84. I tried all kinds of ways to keep from having babies--but each time I slipped up. (39T, an informant who has had twelve pregnancies followed this time by a hysterectomy.)

B. Symptoms of Pregnancy

Most of the symptoms of pregnancy's earliest stages are considered earlier, as signs, even though there is implicit in them a notion of causality--that is, the signs are caused by the fact of pregnancy. The reason for classifying them as signs is, of course, that they function as such--they are used to recognize the woman's condition and predict the arrival of a child, usually very early in the course of gestation.

Other symptoms appear rather later, and have nothing to do with detection of the pregnant state, in the informants' view. Thus the beliefs in the present category have nothing to do with prediction. They are merely accompaniments to one's condition, or things to which one is peculiarly vulnerable at this time.

Food whims are, of course, a classic and culturally validated symptom of pregnancy in many parts of the world. So widespread is the notion that women are apt to want exotic or peculiar foods when they are with child that one may even speculate that there is some physiological basis for the phenomenon, such as vitamin deficiency or anemia, which may produce "cravings" in a large percentage of pregnant women. The requirement that such whims be satisfied if at all possible is also a very widespread cultural phenomenon--perhaps based on the need to give women who are pregnant high priority when it comes to distribution of the available food supply, if they are to bear children who will live to increase and perpetuate the group.

One phenomenon which appears markedly among this particular group of informants, however, has to do with the symptom, sometimes present at other times, but most prevalent during pregnancy, of eating things which are not considered foods by either cultural or medical standards. The habit of eating such "unnatural" substances as clay, plaster, and laundry starch is clinically known as "pica" and known to cultural anthropologists as "geophagy" (earth-eating) from the form it generally takes when found among primitives. The phenomenon is mainly prevalent among women and children wherever it is found in the world--especially among parturient women "who live in impoverished areas, both in the United States and in so-called under-developed nations . . . (It) is frequently associated with iron-deficiency anemia."[8] Recent research has established a causal relationship between this habit of eating alkaline substances and the failure to absorb iron from the diet. It is not yet established that this has an adverse effect upon unborn children, but it certainly makes the mother anemic and may also cause anemia of a chronic type in the fetus.[9] It is also true, however, that some of the clays eaten (in Florida, for example) appear to be iron-rich, so that the clay-eating habit may be adaptive in some areas of the world.

About a third of my informants admitted to eating such substances as are mentioned above, if not with this pregnancy then with some previous one. Several more spoke of relatives who had the habit, and I sometimes suspected that this was a blind for their own indulgence. Besides the most common substances--laundry starch and clay pellets (sometimes imported from the South)--a whole list of other non-foods were reported as having been eaten by my informants, either when they were pregnant or in childhood: Alka Seltzer tablets (undissolved, and chewed up so that they foamed in the mouth), baking soda (beyond the quantity needed to treat heartburn), milk of magnesia in cake form (which I never knew existed), mortar, the dust from soft red bricks, cigarette ashes, and "dirt right out of the window box." The reason always given for eating such substances was that they "just tasked good" or that "I just wanted something gritty (or dry) in my mouth."

85. I've heard that it's bad to eat starch, because it dries up your blood, or something like that. (8T, whose sister ate it, 41T, 33T, and 16R--who defiantly announced, however, that even though doctors say it's bad for you "I don't pay them no mind. I do as I please, and it never hurt me."

86. You aren't supposed to eat a lot of salt when you're pregnant. The doctors don't like it, because it makes you fat. (11P was the only informant who gave a reason for the prohibition. Most other informants knew it was "bad" but if they craved salty things ate them anyway.)

87. I carried my baby lopsided, so I couldn't tell whether it was going to be a boy or a girl. That's because I carried my other baby around so much while I was pregnant. (26T, who added "a woman has no business to carry and lift another child when she's pregnant.")

88. I guess I just got a double dose of everything this time, because it was twins. (5H, who was discussing the discomforts of pregnancy, such as heartburn, swelling feet, and nausea.)

89. If you don't drink enough water when you're pregnant, you're liable to get kidney trouble. (31T, who had it, says the doctors told her this.)

90. If a baby has lots of hair, that will cause the mother to have a lot of gas while she's pregnant. (13T, 40P)

91. I ate so many peaches that first time . . . they had to stop me from it because I was breaking out all over. (40T, who added that her daughter, consequently, "can't eat peaches till this day, either.")

92. When you're pregnant, you likes to eat a whole lot of things you never eats any other time. (42T, who listed among other things, lemon peel soaked in koolade, and vegetables which she usually dislikes. 40T also ate lemon peel, and was the woman who craved cigarette ashes violently. She didn't smoke, but used to buy cigarettes and burn them down to ashes, then eat the ashes with a spoon. Innumerable other strange and not-so-strange food whims were reported, even by women who said they had never had any themselves. The phenomenon is universally known.)

C. Causes Related to Premature Birth and Miscarriage

Prematurity is a long-standing problem among the Negro poor, according to hospital authorities. The precise statistics are not immediately available to me for the hospital ward population at large, but in my own group of fifty informants there were ten whose current baby was premature (i.e., born before the thirty-sixth week, or weighing under five pounds, or both.) Only one of these infants died, and this was an anacephalic child who could not have survived even at full term. In addition to this very high percentage of prematures, there were many mothers who had borne premature babies at another time, and several who had histories of miscarriages.

Since premature infants are more fragile than others, it is safe to assume that the high mortality rate among American Negro infants is, to some extent, associated with the high incidence of prematurity. Without question, both prematurity and infant mortality in the United States show a strong association with low income, regardless of race. (Irelan, 1967:54). The reasons for this are not entirely clear. They are most likely related primarily to general levels of maternal health in the physical sense of the word--but there are those who suspect that there may be a correlation with emotional health as well, i.e., with the degree to which a mother accepts or rejects the idea of having another child. There is even some suspicion among people who have dealt over long periods with the group of mothers from which my informants come that some mothers (especially the youngest ones) induce labor early by various means in order to be rid of the burden of carrying their babies to term.[10]

93. A miscarriage is one of the worst things there is. I know, because my mother told me about the one she had . . . It's better to go ahead and have the baby. (11T.

The ellipsis represents a long and gory tale of anguish. This informant had at first hoped that she would miscarry, because she had given birth four times in as many years.)

94. If you fall, like down the stairs, when you're pregnant, you might start in labor. (7T, who had had such a fall just before she delivered.)

95. If you does a lot of heavy work while you is pregnant, you might cause yourself to have a miscarriage. (20T, who had one a year before, which she attributes to doing heavy factory work and 7T, who cautioned against lifting and straining. Some women, however, denied this was true, since they had worked hard all through their pregnancies with no ill effect.)

96. I didn't lose so much blood (with a miscarriage). I guess I didn't have too much blood. (20T)

97. The night I started in to labor I ate two sour pickles and a dish of collard greens, and that did it. My neighbor next door, she warned me that eating all that would start me in to labor. (27T, who delivered early.)

98. They say when you're pregnant you shouldn't do things like go to the shore, or get out and have a good time, or the baby will come before time. (17P, a teenager who had resented these restrictions, and finally went off to Atlantic City, following which trip she did deliver prematurely.)

99. My first two babies were born in the eighth month, but the last two were full term. I figure the cigarette ashes made me carry the last two longer, so maybe it was a good thing to do. (40P, whose husband and family objected to her strange habit of eating ashes, and who therefore came up with this post facto rationalization. Her first child was born when she was seventeen.

D. Causes of Traits in the Unborn

Prenatal influences are, by far, considered to be the most important cause of peculiar physical or emotional traits in babies. Beliefs regarding the ways in which babies can be "marked" during the mother's pregnancy are more widespread than any others. The idea of heredity is largely relegated to the category of beliefs which deals with specific resemblances between babies and older people related to them--but individualized qualities, whether mental or physical, are usually attributed to some event which occurred before birth.

A baby may be "marked," quite literally, with a blemish or birthmark. But he can also be "marked" psychologically, with a preference or an aversion for something his mother liked or indulged in, and he can be seriously "marked" with physical or mental defect. In most beliefs concerning prenatal influences there are, implicitly, quasi-magical forces at work which emphasize the identity between mother and child --what Frazer once dubbed "sympathetic magic." Generally the child will carry a mark resembling something which affected the mother strongly at some time during her pregnancy.

Newman, in commenting upon beliefs of this nature, points out that

> it is clear that neither the form, implication or content of these beliefs was transmitted by a doctor, nor probably by a written source . . . (they) are evidently a form of ritual behavior using stylized communication, and effecting role validation of both the speaker and the one spoken to. (1965: 136-137)

Such beliefs are generally transmitted by older family members and other women.

Both Newman (1965:140) and Eddington (1968:text #2) have observed that there is, among lower-class Negro women, a tradition which involves the telling of "scare stories" to pregnant women, and that these function as a kind of initiation rite marking the transition to adult status. Many of the memorates which accompanied the beliefs in this collection fall into precisely this category, often being told with much fearsome detail and with great apparent relish.

Newman, in discussing prenatal influences and the ritual function of the transmission of such beliefs, doubts that there is any great expectation that they will "be believed in any very realistic sense (i.e., there may be little or nothing in the way of direct behavioral results)" (Op. cit.:139) My own finding is rather different, based upon the four-point scale I have been using to indicate the level to which an item is actually believed. If the testimony of memorates means anything, one must assume that there is a fairly high level of belief in prenatal influences--by far the greater number of my informants indicated partial or total conviction that various marks of both physical and mental varieties were, indeed, due to something they had done. This did not prevent the causative acts involved--perhaps because the consequences were not deemed serious enough to inhibit self-indulgence.

Of course, nearly all beliefs referring to "marking" are of a type which contains an implicit "control." One can avoid the mark that will be produced by the mother's craving, even if the desire itself is uncontrollable, by satisfying her wishes (or, conversely, by forbidding her unbridled indulgence past a certain point, as it is sometimes stated.) One doesn't have to laugh at anyone, or watch horror movies, or attend funerals. In a few cases, however, the influence which will mark the baby is some surprising and fortuitous event--and in these cases it seems that with the "control" factor lacking the mothers, even if they scoff at such beliefs, may feel some real anxiety. One woman who had seen several sights which violently revolted and frightened her while she was pregnant was in terror that her child would be born deformed in some hideous way. Since she was confined to bed and didn't see the baby for several days, she became quite agitated about it--even though everyone who had seen the baby, including her own eldest daughted, told her it was fine. Another who had had several horrible dreams shortly before delivery was in the same state until she had a chance to reassure herself by being taken to the nursery window to see her child.

Since most of the beliefs which follow also imply control, perhaps they should have been placed in that class of items. Still, there is a kind of organic unity to them all, and since all are not controllable I have placed them together except in those instances where the control was explicitly stated.

100. If you crave something when you're pregnant and you don't get it, and then you touch your body--like if you touch your face--where you put your hand there'll be a mark on the baby, and it will look like the thing you craved. (6H, who had no cravings in pregnancy, anyhow. 31T, who said that her son had a steak on his leg, and knows a little girl with chocolate ice cream all over her face. 32P, 27P, 46P, who says her daughter has a mark that's "either vanilla ice cream or a piece of turkey." She got the first, but "must not have got any turkey, so I guess it's that." Another child of hers has a "black jelly bean right on her behind--and she won't eat no black jelly beans, either." 34T and 2H both maintained that they had heard that there would be both a physical mark on the baby, and that "he'll always want that food you craved all through his life." 32T, my oldest informant, claimed that her husband has a mark shaped like an oyster, and that he has craved oysters all through his life, from which she deduces that his mother wanted oysters.)

101. If you crave something when you're pregnant, and you eats a lot of it, when the baby is born it will have a mark that looks like the thing you craved. (2P and 9P gave this variant of the marking belief above. Testimony was supplied by 40T whose baby had a mark like a hamburger because "the whole time I was pregnant I didn't eat nothin' but hamburgers." This informant's previous child had a steak on his leg, and another child has an allergy to peaches because she gorged on them until she broke out in a rash [see #89]. 49T and 50T both craved hoagies and interpreted small brown marks of uncertain shape as looking "just like a hoagie." The former of these two, however--unbothered by considerations of logical consistency--told me that one daughter of hers with whose pregnancy she wanted hoagies also, "won't have anything to do with them things!" while on the other hand a son with whose pregnancy she loved to eat watermelon and poundcake "just wants to eat them all the time.")

102. If you're born in the winter, that will cause you to be cold-natured all your life. (9T, who says she wears two or three sweaters in the house until well into summer because she was born in winter.)

103. If a baby is born in the summer, like I was, it will sweat all the time. (10T, which is, of course, the converse of the belief directly above, and occurred in the same session.)

104. Things that happen to you while you're pregnant can definitely mark the baby. (24T, who declined to illustrate, but looked grave about it.)

105. Maybe that's why this baby is sucking his finger--because I used to get upset when my sister-in-law's kids would do it in my house. (49P)

106. I guess the reason my baby won't eat is I didn't want anything to eat the whole time I was pregnant with him. (31P, also 1P, whose mother predicted that her baby would "rock after it was born, because I was always rocking.")

107. All the time I was pregnant I was scared I'd see something that would scare me, and it would mark the baby. (48P, who added, however, "My friend told me it was silly--if I was to believe all that stuff I'd be afraid to leave the house the whole time.")

108. My grandmother says her son looks like a chicken. She says that's because when she was pregnant she went into the barn one day and got scared by a chicken, and that's how he got that way. (36H, who added laughingly, "He don't think he looks like a chicken, though--he thinks he looks just fine!")

109. A whole lot of funny things happened to scare me when I was pregnant. A couple of times I just hollered, I was so scared. You're not supposed to touch your face, or it'll mark the baby's face, if something scares you like that. (46T, whose cat aborted and dragged its dead kittens to her feet. Later on she "went to see a two-headed man at the amusement park" [evidently a set of Siamese twins], then still later a nest full of baby robins fell from a tree and were smashed right in front of her. This is the woman who experienced such anxiety when she couldn't see her baby immediately, because she was bedbound.)

110. It's newsy--just like I was the whole time I was pregnant. (25P, referring to her newborn boy, who had just lifted his head up and looked around the room with an alert expression on his face.")

111. If you touch or scratch yourself on your face--or anyplace on your body--while you're pregnant, the baby will have a mark. (2H whose grandmother lived with her, and was constantly cautioning her about this.)

112. You shouldn't call people names when you're pregnant, you'll mark the child. (50T, who prefaced this remark with a story. "With the baby before this one I used to fight with my husband and call him a knotty-headed old hard-headed somthing. And that's the child that won't let you touch her head to comb it. And she <u>do</u> have a knotty head; you can't comb that hair without pulling it, and it hurts her. My mother says it's my own fault because I called her father that.")

113. If you eats a lot of fish and pray hard, your baby will be smart. (9P, who had this from "a lady who is an elder in my congregation.")

114. When you're pregnant you should be careful never to laugh at anybody who's crippled--or at anybody at all, for that matter--or else your child will be born to look like that person. (27P, 36P)

115. My two little girls hung on me the whole time I was pregnant. When they do that, it means they're putting a mark on the baby to make it a girl. (36T, who knew she'd have another girl for this reason.)

116. If you see anything to scare you or make you said, it will mark the baby. (36H, whose grandmother cautioned her not to watch horror movies or attend funerals. She ignored the prohibition, thinking it "old fashioned.")

E. Causes of Distress or Accidents During Labor

Although several investigators have commented on the fact that "scare stories" told to pregnant girls result in terror about delivery, I cannot say that my own findings bore out this contention. (Cf. Eddington, op. cit. and Newman, op. cit., pp. 140) The single exception was the informant who supplied #123. Although such stories were told to me on the ward, and reported by girls to whom they had been told, I never sensed that my informants made any more fuss, or dwelled any more on the pain of delivery than any other group of women I have known. The only specific fear mentioned by an informant was not of the pain of childbirth, but of the examination for pregnancy at clinic. ("My sister told me they shoves something up inside you, and it hurts! She was right, too.") Several of the older women remembered being "scared that first time"--and it is probable that this feeling is not confined to lower-class women or to Negro women. Of course, it is possible that, since most of my informants had already delivered, their fears were no longer in the forefront of consciousness. Nevertheless, I didn't detect excessive worry about delivery in their tales of the delivery room, nor in the folk beliefs themselves. With few and minor exceptions such difficulties as were cited or anticipated during labor were based on realistic factors, not on occult notions, and fears for the baby's welfare were more prominent than fears for their own survival in delivery.

117. If you gets too fat when you're pregnant, you might get far around your heart, and when it's time to have it, they'll have to go looking for that baby. (14T, who referred to an immensely fat patient then in the hospital. 16T agreed that being too fat would give you a "hard time.")

118. If you eat starch, it makes the baby stick to you. (4T, who cited the case of her sister-in-law, who "ate a whole box a day for three months, and when it came time for the baby to be born they had to cut her open to get it out, because it was stuck up inside her.")

119. If you moves when they give you that saddle block, you could end up being paralyzed for life. (4T, referring to spinal anaesthesia.)

120. When a saddle block doesn't work on you it's because you probably moved when they was giving you the needle. (4T)

121. A dry birth is always harder and more painful. (36T, whose membranes had ruptured prematurely so that she had a "dry birth.")

122. I knew my baby would come before they could give me the spinal. I tried to hold it back, but it just popped out while I was lying on my side, 'cause it was in a hurry! (15T, who added that it was lucky the baby was a preemie, weighing under 5 pounds, because "a bigger baby would have tore me all up, coming fast that way.")

123. When I was pregnant the first time, people told me: "When you have a baby you're going to have a whole lot of pain--might even die!" (13T)

124. Another thing is when the doctors comes and examines you in the middle of a

labor pain--and that hurts! (49T)

125. The worst pain was from the baby pressing on my bladder, so I felt like I had to urinate all the time. (49T, who added "but when I tried there wasn't nothing there.")

126. If you do a lot of walking right at the end they say that might bring on your labor. (22H, who was referring to women at full term, but didn't think this was true, since she had walked around a great deal and nothing happened. Her own labor, she says, was brought on by rough play with her little brother, which "caused my water to break.")

127. It's bad to get as nervous as I was. I used to get spells of shakin'--even on the delivery table. I think that made my labor longer. (31T, whose nervousness was not a result of fear of labor, but because she had three small children without a father, and was worried as to how she would manage to support another.)

F. Causes of Resemblances, Genetic Factors

Of course my informants were aware of traits that "run in families" and had the standard American conceptions about such things. (Cf. Schneider, 1968:25 on relations of "blood" in American culture.)

A very curious phenomenon which I observed, however, was the rarity with which mothers referred to resemblances between their new babies and themselves or others in the family. Only two women spontaneously volunteered that the baby "looks just like her uncle--and I couldn't stand him the whole time I was pregnant!" or "this one looks like her brother and her father." When I asked who the baby looked like, of course, there was usually some real or fancied resemblance brought to mind--but it struck me as odd that these ideas were so seldom volunteered, and had to be elicited. A question like "Well, what do you think of your baby?" brought various expressions of pride and satisfaction, but no mention of family resemblance, as I believe it would have among my own friends.

It has been suggested to me that this may result from the fact that the identification of the mother with her child is so strong that there is no need to assert in this fashion that he belongs to her--and that, in fact, this need is more likely to be felt by the father or the grandparents, whose claims must be staked out early. I cannot be sure.

There is quite another kind of "resemblance," however, which may be somewhat distinctive for this group of women. This is the similarity often observed between their own symptoms and those of the baby's father. This phenomenon has been observed in other parts of the United States, usually in rural areas, and has sometimes been compared to the couvade which is known for a number of tribal societies. It differs from the true couvade, however, in that there is no ritual requirement that men experience the symptoms of the women they have impregnated, and in that the symptoms are felt as "real"--that is, they are not part of a set imitative procedure, but are felt as genuine malaise, pain, or other female symptoms.

Wayland Hand suggests that such phenomena, or the expectation of them as normal, serve to "emphasize the sympathetic connection between husband and wife during the ordeal of pregnancy and childbirth." (1957) I would submit that the emphasis on this connection puts this phenomenon in American life quite out of the class of couvade practices elsewhere, for there the idea seems to be to emphasize the equivalent importance of paternity and maternity, rather than the sympathy a man has for his mate. A husband who actually sickens on his wife's behalf is acting quite differently from the one who ritually pretends to labor in order to call attention to his otherwise nonessential role in the birth process. On the other hand, one might conceive of a husband's sympathetic symptoms as expressing an unconscious need to assert his paternity which is otherwise difficult to verify beyond question.

128. Children will usually take after somebody in the family. (14T, who emphasized body build, and cited the fact that one of her daughters is "big-boned, like me, but the baby is short and fat like my mother." 17T, who saw features in her baby which resembled the baby's father, brother and sister, and 46T, who observed that resemblances can take distorted forms, for with one child "I was most ashamed to take that baby home, she looked so bad! She looked like her father--but she was so _ugly!_" Also 13T, whose baby looked like a "brother-in-law--and I couldn't stand him the whole time I was pregnant!")

129. Twins run in families. If either you or your husband is one of twins, there's a good chance of you having them. (32T, whose husband is one of twins. In agreement with the first part of the statement are 30T, 17T, and 39T, all of whom have had twins and cite some family history of twin births.)

130. I'm one of ten children, my father was one of thirteen, and my aunt (that's my father's sister has twenty-one kids. I guess that's why I've got so many. Some of my brothers and sisters has nine and ten kids--I've got eleven. I think it runs in families. (46T)

131. It's the father that makes the baby one sex or the other. (23T, who was disappointed at having a fourth boy, but says "my husband warned me I couldn't get nothing but boys from him!" She had actually given birth to two girls before she was married, but they had a different father and were being raised by her mother. She wanted a "girl to raise by myself," as these older children hardly felt like her own.)

132. If a woman is pregnant, sometimes her husband will get her symptoms. (26T, whose common-law husband was constantly hungry and gained weight while she was pregnant, and suffered low back pains while she was in labor--even though he was at work and didn't know she was in the hospital. These stopped around the time she delivered. 24T, who had heard of men suffering morning sickness and labor pains, 42T, and 49T, whose husband had morning sickness "while all the time _I_ was feeling fine!" Also 46T, who described her brother's food cravings, which matched those of his pregnant girlfriend. "He eats all them things right along with her . . . Look like _he's_ carrying the baby, too!")

G. Causes of Postpartum Symptoms

These were actually little mentioned, and when they were it was not in the explicit or implicit form of a belief, but rather as a complaint of some sort--usually about "afterpains"--and in connection with some measure to relieve the complaint, which classes them as "controls." Only the following, therefore, fit in here, and one is connected with the matter of breast-feeding--which is, of course, a postpartum situation, though not precisely a symptom, perhaps.

It might be noted that very few of my informants breast-feed. Only two were doing so at the time I interviewed them, and only three or four more had ever done so. Of those who had done so and decided against it this time, the reason given was preference for bottle-feeding. (One woman very frankly said "I didn't like having a baby sucking on my titty!")

133. I had a lot of pain earlier this morning because I had some big clots that wouldn't come down. (49T, who added "I should have kept my mouth shut about it, though, because when I told the nurse, sure enough here come the doctor with a glove!")

134. Toward the end of my pregnancies I couldn't hardly sleep at all . . . I guess that's why once the baby is here I sleeps so good--to get caught up, I guess. (46T, who said she doesn't even hear her babies cry at night, after she gets home.)

135. Breast-feeding will spoil your shape, they all say nowadays. (32P, who accounts in this way for the fact that it has gone "out of style" among the younger women. She is 42, and nursed her older children, but was glad to give it up in recent years, even though she believes "it's the best thing for the baby.")

H. Causes of Harm to Babies, and Child Development

Some of the items in this category are prenatal events, some part of early infant care, and almost all--like the beliefs in prenatal influences of the "marking" variety--implicitly contain an element of control. Since, however, the focus is on causality with reference to proper concern for the baby's welfare, they are placed here.

The consequences of failing to act in accordance with these beliefs ("It's bad luck to buy clothes . . ." or "Don't hang curtains . . .") are more serious than the consequences of neglecting to follow beliefs about "marking." They involve the infant's very survival or his generally healthy development, rather than just a minor blemish or small eccentricity of behavior. Those women who really believed in them --either at the total or partial level--tended therefore to observe the implicit prescriptions involved.

The major exception to this rule seemed to be breast feeding, which many people agreed was best for the baby, but which few mothers followed through.

136. It's bad luck to buy clothes before the baby's born--it might even make it be

born dead. (13P, 25P, 23T, 10P, who didn't know what the consequence might be, actually, but said "I'm just scared to do it, that's all." It is, however, permissable for others to buy things ahead of time for the baby, and to give them to the mother at baby showers.)

137. If you hang curtains, or reach and stretch a lot when you're pregnant, the baby might get strangled by the cord. (1H, 31P, 50R, who called this an "old superstition" and added "As hard as I done worked with all of my pregnancies I never had that happen to a one of my (eight) children." 5T, on the other hand, had given birth to a stillborn one year ago who actually had been born with the cord "wrapped twice around its neck" and says that the doctor at Germantown Hospital "told me it must have strangled because I reached up too much while I was pregnant . . . He said it must have been something like that, because he didn't see how the cord would have gotten extended like that otherwise." The patient reports having suffered a deep depression following the events she described.)

138. The infection I had last time caused my baby to have some damage to his brain. (32T, who added, "The same thing happened this time, and I'm so afraid this baby'll be like that, too." The six year old who is brain damaged is a retarded child.)

139. If you eats a whole lot of starch while you're pregnant, the baby will be born with a whole lot of white stuff all over its skin. ('3T, who said that she had eaten three or four boxes of Argo a day with her previous pregnancy, and that her baby was born this way. 6H had been told a similar tale by her sister, but didn't believe it.)

140. If a child gets dropped when it's small, that could maybe cause him to get epilettic (sic) fits later on. (20T, whose son had died at the age of three during a severe epileptic seizure.)

141. If a man beats you when you're pregnant he could hurt you <u>and</u> the baby. (12T, whose husband had beaten her badly before she was hospitalized, and who had not yet delivered. She was concerned that some harm had been done to the unborn child.)

142. If a baby is born with asthma, she'll have it all her life. (14P, who had heard this from other women, and was worried because her 11 month old child at home had asthma.)

143. My baby at home is only eleven months old, and she weighs 33 pounds. The doctor says I kept her on Similac too long, that's why she gained so much weight. He says that's why she isn't walking yet--because she's so fat. (36T)

144. If you take the baby out in the night air you'll give him wind colic. (32H, whose mother told her this, but she observes that "young girls nowadays take their babies out at all hours, and it doesn't seem to hurt them any. I used to follow it when I was young, though.")

145. If a woman drinks too much then them cruelty people will come and take her children away from her. (7T, who confessed that she used to drink heavily, but hasn't had a drop for two years, because a friend's children were taken away and she

was afraid hers would be, too. "Besides," she added, "children ain't going to have no respect for a mother that stays drunk all the time.")

146. If the mother gives a baby away (for adoption) people'd have to think it wasn't no good, and whoever got it would just treat it like a puppy nobody wanted. (20T, who expressed strong disapproval of her sixteen year old roommate, whose baby was being put up for adoption.)

147. If you rock a child to sleep, it'll spoil him. (7T)

148. If you holds a child and loves it too much, it'll get spoiled. (20T, 46T, who said it took her four babies to learn this lesson, 50T, who declared that all seven of hers were spoiled because she always "gave them lots of attention.")

149. If you leave a baby on the bottle too long you'll spoil him. (7T)

150. The baby puts most of its weight on the last two months. That's when you gets large. (5T, who remained small until then, but became so large at the end of her pregnancy that twins were suspected.)

151. They say mother's milk is the best thing for babies. (32T, 9T, 30T, 20T, all of whom were bottle feeding and expressed dislike of nursing. 29T was nursing her baby, as was 7T. 40T expressed regret that she couldn't do so because her "milk wasn't no good" and said the doctors told her at clinic that she "wouldn't be able to do it this time, either." Later, however, she expressed revulsion at the idea--likely the real reason for not nursing in this case, too.)

152. Small babies grow faster than large babies, because they got to catch up. Sometimes they even grow bigger than the ones that was born big. (9T, who had had a premature baby before this one.)

153. Even after they're born, boys is lazier than girls. That's why they say a boy is harder to train, because they're lazier than girls. (36T)

I. Causes of Miscellaneous Effects

154. I got my first gray hairs from this baby, 'cause I was worried to death about having another baby. That's because I had so much trouble with my last one. (32T, who is 42 years old, and has a six year old retarded boy--the last before this child.)

155. It's bad, having babies too fast. It can give you cancer, and if it don't give you that it can still ruin your health. (13T, who is 32 years old and had three children in three years after many years of barrenness. She requested and got a tubal ligation this time. See also belief #69, in which she accounts for her sudden fertility.)

156. Every cake I tried to bake while I was pregnant would fall, or be wet in the center, or something would go wrong with it. I figure it was because I was pregnant, because the rest of the time I bakes real good. (46T, who intended to test her theory

by baking something as soon as she got out of the hospital to see if it would now rise. This belief is rather closely related to #206 in that there is a notion that the influence of a pregnant or bleeding woman might contaminate food in some fashion.)

157. In those days (when grandmother bore her children, in rural Virginia) they didn't give a woman no help and no pity. Two, three days after the baby was born she was back in the fields working again like nothing had happened. If you were weak, you died. (36T)

158. A person could kill themselves by trying to get rid of their baby. (25T, who believes, however, that it is not a police matter unless someone else performs the operation. Also 20T).

159. If you're pregnant it's better to go on and have it. If you try to get rid of it, you could get sick, or even bleed to death--or if it don't work you might hurt the baby. (1T)

160. If you get rid of any babies in your lifetime, then when you're on your deathbed those babies' souls will come and scream at you that you is a murderer. (34H, whose mother told her this, but who thinks it's superstitious nonsense.)

III. CONTROLS

A. Controls Over Conception

This is a straightforwardly "modern" category of beliefs, almost without exception. Only two informants came up with the contraceptive lore of an earlier day when women hoped that prolonged nursing or douching after intercourse would help them to avoid pregnancy.

There is an interesting "time gap" noticeable here, however, between the really pre-scientific methods just mentioned and the recent advances represented by The Pill and the intrauterine device, or "coil." Only one informant ever mentioned that former standby of the first scientific birth-control crusaders, the diaphragm--which until this decade was widely used throughout the world by the middle classes interested in limiting their families. This was, it would seem, an era that completely passed over women of the lower classes, leaving practically no mark--and one must suppose that this was due to the general lack of educational programs affecting these women, in a period when physicians generally disseminated such information only to their private patients. Thus until very recent legislation, which was passed only after the age of Pills and IUD's had arrived, women of the ghetto population were unlikely to have much recourse save prayer, or the rather unreliable condom. The latter, in any case, depended on male cooperation which was not always forthcoming.

The Pill and the IUD are touted both in the educational program at Temple and among the women themselves as being by far the most reliable contraceptive methods short of tubal ligation, and were those most often mentioned. A very few women advocated the use of vaginal foams, usually because they had heard of side-effects of the two most certain methods in general use, and were afraid to use them. (This was, incidentally, the reason given by the lone, conservative diaphragm user as well.) Condoms were looked upon only as an emergency measure for young girls to use with their boyfriends if they were inexperienced and had made no other preparation. Vaginal foams, for which no prescription is needed, were sometimes advocated for the same sort of contingency. Pills, of course, are a prescription drug and seldom were obtained before the first pregnancy. The IUD, since it must be inserted by a physician, fell into the same category.

It is probable that, in a population in which large families are both common and traditional, the point at which families are really felt to be too large is somewhat higher than for middle class groups. (One informant felt that four children was a small family--which in relative terms was the truth, since her mother had had no less than eleven. Few married informants meant to stop having babies before they had at least three.) There is no doubt, however, that once this point is reached, at whatever number of children seems reasonable to the mother, there is real gratitude for means to avoid further pregnancies--and firm intentions to take advantage of the autonomy they bestow, even when the intention is not always carried out.

Some women referred to husbands or boyfriends who objected to their use of birth control techniques--whether or not they interfered with pleasure. The attitude usually expressed was that they intended to use them anyway--sometimes without the man's knowledge. "What he don't know won't hurt him," said several women, then added "He's not the one that's got to have them." ("And if men did have to, there wouldn't be any babies in the world at all!" said one girl.)

161. Down home they believes that nursing the baby will keep you from getting pregnant again--that you can't get pregnant until after you stops nursing. (50P, who cited the case of an aunt who nursed all her children for two years, and "every one of them was born two years and nine months apart." The informant, however, preferred not to nurse her babies, and therefore didn't rely on this method.)

162. When I told my mother after my first intercourse, she taught me how to douche after intercourse to keep from getting pregnant. (11R, who now knew that she was lucky indeed not to have become pregnant using this technique, and since tried the pill but had bad side effects, and intended to try the IUD next time.)

163. Some parents, when they wants to keep a daughter from having babies when they isn't married, has them spayzed (sic) like a dog. (20T actually believed this--it is part of the folklore "down home in Mississippi," as is a tale of a mother who slept in the room with her daughter "and kept her hand on the girl's privates the whole night to keep any boys from getting to her!")

164. If you do something with a boy, you should at least protect yourself with something you buy at the drugstore for the boy to use. (3T was referring to condoms, which her mother had told her about "a long time ago." She was seventeen and had just had her first child.)

165. When the man uses protection, it's not a safe method to keep you from getting pregnant. (30T)

166. When you uses the foam, you puts it up there two or three hours before you has a relationship, then you can use a Lysol douche several hours later. (17T)

167. Emco (a foam) will keep you from getting pregnant as long as you remember to use it. (19T)

168. The pills sometimes can help somebody that can't have children. They're supposed to add something that maybe you didn't have before, and that was why you couldn't have no children. (36T, who knew a girl, she said, who was given pills to regulate her menstrual cycle, following which, as soon as she discontinued them, she conceived.)

169. If the pill don't work, I'll get me a coil, and if that don't work, I'll get myself tied up like that lady across the hall. (25T, who had just endured a very difficult labor, and was determined not to chance more than another two, it would seem.)

170. If you really takes them the way they tells you to, the pill will always keep you from getting pregnant. (34T, 8T, 25T. This belief was, of course, implicitly stated many more times--but usually negatively in terms of failure to take them and ending up pregnant. See Causes of Pregnancy.)

171. If you have your tubes tied, you don't ever have to worry about having any more babies. (13T, 14T, both of whom had done so. 1T, 2T, 34T)

172. If you keeps away from boys--that's the only sure way not to have any more. (22T, age sixteen, who had just had her second child, and now declared her intention of following her own advice.)

173. A coil has less side effects than the pill, so I'd rather take that to keep from having any more babies right away. (36T)

174. A coil is supposed to keep you from having any more babies if you don't want them. (23P, 31P, 36T, who had three children and said "I just refuse to have any more babies.")

175. If you can't take the pill, the next best thing is a coil. (11T, who added that she was going to use Emco foam besides, "because this time I'm not taking any chances.")

176. If you ever had a cyst, or either a tumor, they tells you not to use the pills. It could cause cancer. Then you got to get a coil. (9P, who had once had a tumor removed, and been told this by doctors.)

B. Control of Unwanted Pregnancy

In this category are the numerous beliefs and prescriptions for producing abortion--either with or without assistance from others. The practice is morally disapproved, and in addition greatly feared, and no woman interviewed ever admitted to having attempted to produce an abortion in herself or anyone else. There were, however, many women who, after they had come to feel at ease with me, were quite ready to discuss the various methods they had heard of, their relative efficacy, and their possible consequences. Two or three teenage girls seemed to have more lore on this subject than anyone else I encountered--a fact which rather shocked my middle-class soul, I'm afraid, since they were so very young. I tried hard not to show it.

The methods range from perfectly sound ones to some which probably are without effect. The former are usually dangerous in the hands of untrained persons, of course--and most of the latter are probably innocuous, if sometimes unpleasant-tasting brews taken by mouth.

177. I hear tell that there are shots a doctor can give you to start you in labor if you don't want the baby. They cost about $100. (34T)

178. I've heard of women taking a catheter--or a clothes hanger, even, and sticking it up inside their womb to break the water and make the baby come. (29T, who adds that this is dangerous, though, and can cause hemhorrage. Besides, says this informant "When you really think about it, that's murder." 34T, 23T, who had heard of this being done regularly in a New Jersey brothel when prostitutes became pregnant, 27T, who says she'd never risk doing this "because I wants to live!" and 39T, who knows of an eighteen year old girl who has one child, and has aborted three times since by this method because "Her mother told her she better not bring home no more babies after that first one . . . And each and every time she done landed up in the hospital. She's got a lot more nerve than I got!" Also 20T)

179. You can get rid of a baby if somebody beats you across the belly with the flat side of a board. (23T, who had told about the brothel in Jersey, said that this was another method "the man there used to use when one of his girls got caught.")

180. If you drink a whole lot of castor oil, that can get rid of the baby, too. (29T, 34P, 1T, who recommends a dosage: "a whole bottle" and said to follow it with a drink of hot water.)

181. You can get rid of a baby, they say, by taking quinine pills and hot coffee. Then you sit in water as hot as you can stand. (29P)

182. Another way to get rid of a baby is to drink gin with quinine in it. (34P)

183. If you sit in hot water with some mustard in it, they says that will get rid of the baby, if you don't want to be pregnant. (1P, who is fifteen, and knew quite a few recipes for abortion, but was "scared to try it." She was one of fourteen children, and believed that her mother had also performed several abortions on herself, but wasn't sure how she had done it. She remembered one occasion on which her mother had "almost died, she lost so much blood," however.)

184. They say if you sit in a tub of hot water, that will help bring labor on to get rid

of the baby. (34H, who thinks this is nonsense, is herself a practical nurse, and knows better methods.)

185. If a girl wants to get rid of her baby, you should drink some hot water with hot peppers soaked in it. (1P, 34H, 29P, who said "a man once told me this one." This was the only bit of lore which was attributed to a man, except for two sign beliefs which had come from fathers. (See beliefs #7 and #46.)

186. If you drink some sassafras tea, they say that will make you have an abortion. (34H)

187. Gin mixed with hot coffee is one way to get rid of a baby, they say. (29P)

C. Control of Comfort and Health in Pregnancy

As Newman has aptly observed, "If there is anything a pregnant woman knows, it is that when her condition is known, all the world is thereby given license to offer her advice. The large majority of such communications come to the expectant mother from women who have already had children--either older women in the family or others who are or may be complete strangers. It is a time when people are free to speak personally who would not, under normal circumstances, be able to do so." (op. cit.:138)

Much of the advice so offered has to do with the health or comfort of the expectant mother during what is conceived of throughout American culture as a time of discomfort and vulnerability to danger--the latter affecting both mother and child. Many women feel annoyed by the freedom with which such advice is offered, and complain of the "nosiness" of other women at this time in their lives. These are the women, as a rule, who (at least verbally) place their main faith in the advice of doctors, and scoff at most other advice. There are some, however, who seem to enjoy the protectiveness expressed toward them in this manner by older women--especially their mothers. Also, in a very realistic sense, the help of neighbors, friends and relatives can be indispensable among the poor during pregnancy, because they function so close to the margins of existence much of the time. This is especially true when a woman goes into labor and must be taken to the hospital, and her other children looked after for several days. It is worth taking unasked-for advice for a few months to assure that someone will be on call when needed.

188. When I was pregnant I just did what the doctor told me to do. (3T, 4T, were stating an ideal, most likely, rather than describing their actual behavior. These were both girls who expressed some resentment of the interference of older women. Both were teenagers, and evidently experiencing some adolescent revolt as well as the strong emotions of a first pregnancy. "Doctor's advice" probably provided a convenient shield against older women's advice.)

189. When I was pregnant at fifteen, my mother wouldn't even let me take none of that tonic my grandmother used to send up from down South every year. She wouldn't even let me take aspirin! (46P, five of whose eleven illegitimate children had been born while she lived in her parents' house. She gave up this rather atypical degree

of dependency only when the house became so crowded that her parents insisted that she find her own place.)

190. My mother wouldn't let my cousin even come to the house, the first time I was pregnant. She didn't tell me then, but later I found out it was because she was afraid she'd tell me about getting an abortion, 'cause she'd had a whole bunch of them. And my mother told me not to let <u>anybody</u> take me to anyone who said they could get rid of the baby. (46T)

191. A doctor told my sister that she had this craving for starch and baking soda because she had a deficiency in her diet. He gave her iron and vitamins and she lost the craving right after that. (29T)

192. You takes baking soda for heartburn when you're pregnant. (36T, who added, however, that "you got to be careful not to take too much of that stuff, though. Just like starch and all them things, it can be bad for you.")

193. They told me to go on a low-salt diet and they told me to stop drinking lots of soda. (4P, who said these were doctors' instructions for treatment of edema of pregnancy.)

194. The doctors say I should eat lots of red meat and rare liver because my blood is low. (31T, who was quite anemic, but didn't follow the instructions, even though she believed in their efficacy, because she couldn't bear to eat "meat with the blood all running out of it.")

195. If I drank Pepsi or Coke first thing in the morning, it would settle my stomach and keep me from gagging. (36T, whose remedy probably did work, in fact.)

196. When I had cramps near the end of my time I would lie across my husband's belly, and the cramps would go right away. (43T, whose belief in the magical efficacy of her husband's touch was very real.)

D. Control Over the Course of Labor

Whereas most mothers place a good deal of confidence in medical recommendations during pregnancy, labor is rather another matter. Even though hospital delivery is seen as almost indispensible to the safety of mother and child, women are rather ambivalent about the detailed medical management of labor, and quite a few preferred staying home until the last possible moment in order to avoid "them doctors messing you around" during labor. There is a rather strong sense, in this group of informants, that a woman knows how she feels better than anyone else, and should be listened to when she tells the doctor. This is most evident among women who have had several children and are, therefore, experienced with labor and delivery. A sense of her own and the baby's autonomy is very marked here, and interference with this autonomy is viewed with some hostility.

It is interesting to note how this attitude dovetails with the "natural childbirth" ideology of a dozen or more years ago, even though this group of women had never heard of such a thing and it was chiefly in the nature of a fad among educated middle-class people. In this latter group, of course, the ideology of maternal autonomy at birth was a complete break with that of their mothers' generation, who had placed total reliance on medical management and rejected their mothers' "old wives' tales" to the point where they never mentioned them to this generation of young women. (Cf. Newman, 1965:129-30)

Whereas the intellectual middle-class views of "natural childbirth" advocates represent the end of a series of pendulum swings in birth ideology, however, that of my lower-class Negro informants seemed rather to represent a continuous tradition which is rooted in the idea--and the fact--that birth has traditionally been the exclusive province of women among the poor. (Indeed, there were two informants whose first children, born in the South, had been delivered by midwives--and one whose mother had had two babies delivered by a "granny woman" right here in Philadelphia less than seventeen years ago.) Untold generations of black women have had to depend on their own skills and resources in the life-crisis of childbirth, and hospital care is a relatively recent innovation for them. Perhaps that is why there is still present a kind of confidence in self-management which is less characteristic or wholly absent in the more medically privileged segments of the population. (It was, indeed, this self-confidence to which I intuitively appealed in my approach to the informants.)

Female solidarity, of course, is important in this subculture, and has been amply documented. The correlate of this--a certain semi-humorous malice toward males (often enough including doctors as well) emerges which is exemplified by the first belief in this section. This is a technique calculated to show men what labor is like, presumably so that they will have proper respect for the pains of childbirth. Several informants to whom I later recited this particular formula laughed heartily, and said they wished they'd known what to do--because it would have served the baby's father right.

197. If you crawl over your husband three times in the bed while you're pregnant, he'll get your labor pains. (26T, who claims she did this and that her husband did, indeed, suffer her pains. 41H, 42H)

198. It's better to stay home as long as you can when you start in to labor. (7T, who explained that "If you comes in too early the doctors starts messing you around and it makes the pains worse." 30T, who said that "If you can walk around the house you can fight the pains better. When you gets tired of walking you just lie down and roll from side to side." 13T, who agreed with the last informant and, like her, objected to the hospital practice of confining laboring women to bed--though she did agree "that's the safest for the baby." 48T, who told of waiting until the "pains was ten minutes apart" before waking her husband to take her in, and was rather shamefaced that she had "kicked up a fuss" when she arrived at the hospital. 4R also stayed home to walk around, but said "it really didn't help the pain.")

199. The doctor just told me to "take another walk around the block"--they tries to seduce (sic) you in labor that way. (17P)

200. The nurses in the delivery room was nasty, but the doctors they was nice. One of them even offered to hold my hand--but I asked him to rub my belly instead. That helped the pain, too. It reminded me how my husband used to rub my belly when I had cramps while I was pregnant. (33T)

201. Midwives is different from doctors. The main difference is, they don't give you nothing for the pain. Then, too, the midwife asked me to push and strain--I think that's why the baby split my womb in being born. (20T, who added a description of the midwife's technique of having her raise her knees up, then bracing the mother's knees with her back, so that she could push. Later "She reached her hands up in there and pulled the baby out.")

202. Only one of my labors was what you call normal. The baby was born after twelve hours, and I didn't need any shot to bring it on, so that was a normal birth. (14T, who has had seven pregnancies, only four live births, and describes all but one labor as difficult.)

E. Control Over Postpartum Events

The postpartum period is marked by concern for the welfare of both mother and child on the part of those in attendance and on the part of the mother herself. There was little mention made, however, among these informants, of measures concerned with the infant's well being in the delivery room. It seemed that this was viewed firmly as the province of doctors and nurses. Only when something appeared to be going wrong were the activities of the doctor noted and mentioned, as when a baby failed to breathe. In more routine deliveries in which the baby was apparently vigorous the measures taken for its care were either not performed in the mother's presence, or not carefully observed by the mother.

203. I knew they could revive the baby so long as they was getting a heartbeat. First they cleared its mouth and nose of mucous, then they slapped it and tied the cord. When it wasn't crying by that time they sent for a respirator and did mouth-to-mouth respiration on it, and then it began to cry. (17T, who is a former practical nurse, and therefore had the vocabulary to describe exactly what was taking place. 48T, whose baby also failed to breathe right away after being induced because it was well past term, merely said that "the doctors had to work over him for a long time.")

204. Down South the mid-nurse wraps up the afterbirth, then takes it out in the yard and burns it. If you leaves it lying around, something bad is supposed to happen--at least that's what the old people believes. (50P, whose first two children were delivered by South Carolina midwives. 20P reports the same procedure when a midwife delivered her first baby down in Mississippi.)

205. My mother and grandmother always told me "Stay in the bed nine days, rest three days, then feed that baby." (50H, who was forced to follow this postpartum formula for her first two babies, delivered "down home" in South Carolina--but "used to sneak out the bed when nobody wasn't looking," hated being forced to nurse her first two, and abandoned the practice described as soon as she came north to Phila-

delphia, where her remaining six children were born.)

206. Down home they don't let you cook anything till after the (postpartum) bleeding stops. They say you're not clean during that time. If you touch food it will spoil it. (50P, Note the interesting similarity to the belief of a Philadelphia born informant, #156.)

207. An ice bag helps the pain in your breasts when the milk ain't dried up yet. Them pills they gives you don't do anything to dry you up. A binder is good, too--it hurts, but if you takes it off you just runs like anything. (42T)

208. I never wears a binder when my milk is coming in. The one time I wore one of them things, the milk backed all up under my arms and gave me milk boils. It's better to just let it run, then soon it begins to dry up, after they gives you them pills. (46T)

209. You needs to wear a binder around you after you gives birth, to keep your insides in place. (20T, who refers to abdominal binders.)

210. You should have your baby in the hospital, because home ain't sanitary enough. You or the baby could get an infection. (43T, who added "I knows I'm always forgetting to dust.")

211. A heat lamp is good for the pain when you got stitches. (41T, 43T)

212. Aspirin, like they give you here, ain't no good for the afterpains. You needs something stronger to kill <u>those</u> pains. (4T)

F. Control Over Traits of the Unborn and Newborn

There are relatively few positive measures which can be consciously taken to see that the baby is, or will be in future, beautiful or otherwise fortunate. Most of the beliefs about things affecting the baby's fate are phrased as causes rather than controls--although for many of the causes, as has been pointed out earlier, there is an implied control which the mother may exercise if she is conscientious. Negative controls (cursing, for example) are not in the hands of the mother but are a result of malevolence on part of someone else--although the single person who referred to "cursing" seemed to see this as a belief which belongs to another time and place.

Misfortune is a frequent accompaniment to a life of poverty, however, and the misfortunes which fate may inflict on one's offspring are, perhaps, just one more item in the catalogue of troubles that can occur. One woman had a retarded child, and another had a baby who died of "an epilettic (sic) fit" as well as a son whose retardation she had only become aware of after he started school. A third woman had a son who, as a result of a serious fall, was now braindamaged and blind. Their distress and grief was perhaps less hysterical, but was no less real than that which any other mother in our society would express. I had the impression that all three had, far from accepting the situation fatalistically, done their best--often under difficult conditions of long trips and much inconvenience--to get all possible help for their handicapped children.

213. Down South they still believe people can curse the mother, and it will affect the baby she's carrying, if she's pregnant. (2P, who told a tale of such a curse being placed on her aunt, who subsequently bore a child with a nervous ailment which caused him to "bark like a dog all the time, so people wouldn't have anything to do with him.")

214. You should never leave the baby's shoes on top of the dresser, or anyplace high. You ought to always leave them on the floor, or else the baby will be restless. (9T)

215. Down home, when you comes to the house to visit a new baby the first time, you're supposed to put a dime in the baby's hand to give it good luck. (1P, 2H, 9P)

216. The first time the baby goes outside it's not supposed to be the mother that carries it. If she carries it, it's supposed to be bad luck. (11P, who added that the person who does carry the baby is usually a close friend or a relative, someone the mother would like the baby to grow up to be like.)

217. You can shape the baby's nose if you pinch it, and its head by pressing it into the shape you want it to be. (22T, whose grandmother told her this. 20T demonstrated the technique on her own child, explaining that it should be done a few times every day.)

218. If you name the baby for somebody real smart, maybe it'll be smart, too. (41P)

219. I told my husband to go and ask somebody that has girls how they did it, before I'll have another child for him! (33H, who had just had her fourth boy, and complained that her husband "don't know how to make anything but boys." The suggestion was a ribald one, referring to the position used in intercourse.)

G. Control Over Infant Health and Welfare

This section covers, in the main, home remedies used for common complaints of early infancy, with a few that run a bit past that stage and into early childhood. There are two which refer to prenatal precautions to prevent death or harm to the infant. Essentially these same two beliefs are also found under "causes," but these particular informants stated them explicitly in the format of "controls," so they are repeated here. (See #220 and 221)

This fairly large group of items illustrates dramatically the way in which, in this particular genre, one will find new wine in old bottles. Many of the remedies and prescriptions are quite obviously venerable indeed--to the point where probably there are few people in other segments of contemporary American society that have ever heard of them. (Here, again, the relative recency with which modern medical care has become available to even urban poor people is most likely the salient factor, as it was regarding management of labor.) On the other hand, there is a good admixture of modern-day remedies and health measures (hospital circumcision, aspirin, teething lotion) to show graphically how the form of "superstition" may be adapted to new knowledge and techniques. The level of the knowledge itself is not, in essence, much different whether one uses a broth made of asafoetida or aspirin to reduce the baby's fever--though the efficacy of the latter may well be greater. The reason for using the asafoetida <u>or</u> the aspirin doesn't change. It is something which some more or less authoritative person (be it the granny-lady or the doctor) has told one to employ to obtain the desired result.

220. My grandmother told me not never to laugh at anybody, or say anything about them, because if I poked fun at somebody my baby might be born the same way they are. (36P, who added "But I don't like to laugh at people anyways. If somebody has something wrong with them I just feel sorry.")

221. You shouldn't hang curtains when you're pregnant, because the cord will wrap around the baby's neck and strangle it. (17H)

222. If a baby is born with yellow jaundice, they puts it under a blue light, out there in the nursery. (23T, whose baby was in the nursery for this reason.)

223. It's better to have a baby circumcised while it's in the hospital. When a boy is older, they suffers a lot if they has to have it done. (27T, who illustrated the latter part of the statement with a tale of a neighbor's eleven year old's circumcision.)

224. The hospital tells you to give the baby his bottle at room temperature, but it's better--and the baby likes it better--if it's warm. (7T)

225. If the formula is too thin the baby will be hungry no matter how much you give him. (42T, 40T, who added that the hospital formula "hasn't got no body to it. When I get the baby home and put her on my own formula, with Carnation in it, that's got some body to it! They grows real good on that.")

226. If the baby is restless you add a little bit of catnip tea to its bottle. (11T)

227. When my oldest son used to cry in his sleep, they told me the devil was chasin' after him. When I picked him up, though, he'd stop, 'cause I'd drove the devil away. (31P, who expressed scepticism, but still believed in being on the safe side.)

228. You should wipe the new baby's skin with a wet diaper. It makes his skin pretty. (35P, 30T, 36T, 37T, who added that this would "cure a rash if the baby's got one.")

229. Before the naval cord drops off, you clean it with alcohol every time you go to diaper the baby. That keeps it from getting infected. (41T. This was standard practice taught the mothers in the hospital, and followed by nearly all of them.)

230. If you burn the naval cord when it drops off, the baby will never slobber. (37P)

231. When the cord drops off, don't let that stump drop on the floor, or it will make

the baby sick to its stomach, or something like that. (9H, who says this is a belief from "down home" in North Carolina.)

232. For colic my mother used to make my father blow smoke into the mole on top of the baby's head. It's supposed to be good for a baby that's restless at night, too. (11T, who hadn't needed to try it. The "mole" is the fontanel, or soft spot in an infant's skull.)

233. If the baby is colicky, blow some smoke into its milk. (29T)

234. For colic, you gets some gum asafizzity (sic) at the drugstore for thirty-five cents. You soak it in hot water for a few hours, then you take about 1/2 teaspoon of that tea and mix it with an ounce of warm sugar-water and feed it to the baby. It will cure the colic. (26T, who says this worked better than anything the doctors had prescribed at clinic for her first child. The recipe was her mother's. 13T had heard that a broth made of asafoetida was good for colic, but gave no details, as she'd never needed it.)

235. When a baby has hard teething, my mother told me, you slice an onion and put it in the baby's sock. Then you take some alcohol and rub the baby's stomach and rub some sweet niter on its gums, and the next day the baby will feel just fine. The onion draws out the fever. (11T, 22H gave only the part about the onions, but said she wouldn't try it because it would "make the baby's shoes stink.")

236. Sweet niter, that you buys in a little bottle at the drugstore, is good to rub on a baby's gums when he's teething. If he has a fever, you gives him a little bit of it to drink, mixed with sugar water, and it's supposed to bring the fever down. (26T)

237. You shouldn't let a baby chew on any old paper that's lying on the floor. If a baby eats paper it will make his gums hard, so he'll teethe hard. (9T)

238. When the baby is teething, give it a teething ring to chew on, and buy teething lotion at the drugstore to rub its gums with. (15T. Also 22T, who gave only the last part.)

239. Some people hangs a little piece of gum asafizzity (sic) around the baby's neck for teething--to draw out the fever. (26P, who thought the internal use of asafoetida was more likely to work, and objected to the terrible smell of this stuff hung around the neck. 33H)

240. A tea made out of gum asafizzity will draw out the fever if a baby is teething hard. (26T)

241. When a baby is teething hard, you hang an egg in the baby's room, inside an old sock. When the egg dries up so that you can't hear anything inside when you shakes it, the tooth will be through. (22P. Probably quite true. It takes about 2 weeks for an egg to dry out!)

242. For teething, my grandmother told me to catch some sour pigs and put them in a

little cloth bag, and hang it around the baby's neck. (22H, who explained that "sour pigs" are the greyish, fat little maggots found in sour mops and dirty scrub cloths sometimes. She thought this was a revolting idea, and didn't follow the advice. The grandmother was from Virginia.)

243. A mole's foot around the baby's neck will help the baby with teething. You wrap it up in a piece of cloth and hang it on a string around the baby's neck. (20P, whose father told her to do this.)

244. If you hang a dime around the baby's neck on a string it will make teething easy. (37P. The same belief, but using a penny rather than a dime was cited by 9P and 16H. The technique is to drill a hole in a coin and hang it on a chain or string as an amulet.)

245. A piece of gum asafizzity, if you hang it around the baby's neck, is supposed to draw out the fever when the baby has a cold. (26P, 13T, who used a bunch of asafoetida roots instead of the gum form.)

246. They uses asafoetida for making a tea for fever, or else to clean children out. (46P, who added "they gives it to grown people, too, for the high blood pressure.")

247. When the baby has a cold or a fever, you keeps the baby warm, and gives it half a baby aspirin and plenty to drink. (22T)

248. To wean the baby from the breast you gives it a pacifier, and gradually gets it used to a bottle. (20T, who nursed her first two.)

249. If you don't keep little colored girls' hair in braids it'll break off. (20T, who added, "My grandmother used to keep the children's hair in a stocking to make it grow long. I had hair that would wind right around my neck when my grandma was taking care of me.")

250. My mother believed in cod liver oil. She kept a great big bottle in the kitchen, and we all had to take a teaspoonful every morning when we were young. (29H)

251. My grandmother used to send us spring tonic up from the South every year. It was made out of the foot of a cow. It was some kind of oily-base stuff that tasted and smelled real nasty--like the cow had been eating garlic. I don't know how they makes it. They uses it to rub on you too, sometimes. (46H)

252. My mother used to line all eleven of us kids up the first Saturday of every October and give us each a tablespoon of castor oil with a glass of orange juice after it--to keep the cold out during the winter. (29H)

253. The old people down home breaks a child of sucking its thumb or its finger by smearing it with chicken shit. (20R thinks this to be a poor idea since chickens are filthy and might give the child something. "Besides, smart kids used to go right out to the pump and wash the stuff right off.")

254. When I had pneumonia when I was little, my mother gave me a spoonful of sugar

with some kind of oil on it. I don't know what it was, but it broke the fever, and I got well fast after that. (35T)

IV. MISCELLANEA

In this category, I have placed a rather mixed bag of statements which do not obviously fit the three functional categories, but are nevertheless mostly of a stereotypic form which indicates that they are not merely casual utterances.

A handful of these items, in actuality, belong to another genre--one which Honko (1968:13) calls "ficts." These are utterances which are widely used, even though no adult person actually believes them, often for the purpose of answering children's questions on embarrassing subjects such as sex and childbirth. In short, they are the "white lies" which parents have used since time immemorial--not to convey information or knowledge, but to satisfy curiosity without conveying it. Honko suggests, however, that though ficts are known untruths they do serve a function in culture, for "with their help the norms are maintained." (Ibid.) The norms in this case are, presumably, those pertaining to the protection of children from knowledge they are not considered ready for, and the protection of adults from embarrassment in the discussion of "delicate" subjects.

There are also a number of highly stereotyped statements of value included in this miscellaneous category. Such beliefs often have to do with major institutionalized relationships, such as that between husband and wife, or mother and child. Thus one has succinct statements of what is due a husband that it wouldn't be "right" to deny him, (even though it may not please the wife entirely) or what constitutes an "ideal" sort of family or a good or bad relationship within the family. (See beliefs #263-268)

The nature of the sexes and the ways in which stereotypes are applied to boy babies versus girl babies will be commented upon later. Several of the statements which were made apropos this subject are included here for reference, as is one on the matter of bearing twins.

Less obviously stylized utterances are also included here, even though they may belong to no particular genre of folklore, largely because they express in succinct terms very central values and value conflicts which appeared as recurrent themes in my interviews with the informants. I have not attributed these to more than one informant each, since they are non-stereotyped expressions, but they indicate concerns which cropped up more than once in casual fashion, usually in rather diffuse general conversation. Here are expressed certain concerns which will be discussed in the last section of this thesis.

At the very end are three brief statements which have to do with notions of the supernatural element operating in human existence. These, too, will come up for later discussion in terms of the cultural inferences which may be drawn from them.

255. Babies come out of the cabbage patch. They're brought by Mr. Cabbage. (34

was told this as a child.)

256. Babies come from the sky. (13 thought this "until I was a big, grown girl.")

257. The stork brings babies. (40, whose mother told her this, but when babies kept arriving "and I didn't see nothing flying around" she stopped believing it.)

258. Jesus brings the baby. (40 tells her children, ages 2, 3, and 4 this one in preference to the above, which she was told, and defends her use of a fict by saying "In a way, anyhow, it's true. Jesus does make babies get born.")

259. When I was small I believed the doctor brought the baby in his little black bag. (46, whose mother gave birth at home when she was eleven. Also 31, whose grandmother told her this.)

260. When I was young my mother told me babies grow inside the mother's stomach, and the doctor has to cut all along that black line down the middle of your stomach to get them out. (15, who added that there were many neighbors, in the project where she lived, who "were always having babies. I wondered how they would let themselves be cut open all those times, and I figured they'd end up just a mess of scars! I didn't learn the truth until I was in hygiene class in high school." Also 30)

261. My daughters all know that the baby grows inside mom's stomach. (46, who doesn't, however, speak of telling them how the baby gets there.)

262. After I was married my mother told me how babies were really born, but I didn't believe her. I didn't see how anything that size could come out that place! (30, who was married at fourteen in Philadelphia by means of "upping" her age to sixteen.)

263. Pregnancy, unless the baby is premature or something, lasts forty weeks. (1, having her baby at fifteen, was showing off her knowledge. Most women knew this, of course.)

264. They say once you leaves a man, even if you goes back together again, your home life won't never be the same. It will make him feel he's not much of a man, and he'll wonder what you've been up to when you wasn't with him. (41T, whose record indicated that she and her husband were separated, but she denied it. Her roommate, 39T, agreed with this statement, saying "They says it messes up their pride, or something like that.")

265. Every man wants a son. (30T)

266. A man wants a son to carry his name. (31T, 41T put it this way: "You got to give a man a Junior if he wants one. It wouldn't be right not to." She named her baby Cecil, which she hated, because her husband's name is Cecil.)

267. It seems like the men that has the most children likes them the least. The ones that don't have many seems to love children more. (50T, who had eight and complained that their father didn't do anything for them or show them any affection.)

268. There's some things a mother is better at when it comes to taking care of kids. Men just don't know how to do some things. (9T, 29T)

269. A boy and a girl is a rich man's family. (12H)

270. It's no harder having twins than having just one baby--in fact I think it would be fun. (16T, who referred to the labor itself in the first part of her statement, and to the fun of rearing twins only as a kind of afterthought.)

271. If God means you to carry a baby full term, that's what you should do. (29T, expressing moral disapproval of women who seek abortions.)

272. You got to take each child as it comes, and trust the Lord to provide. (20P, who has had two defective children and a stillbirth. 36R says her grandmother expresses sentiments like this, and disapproves of birth control. "She thinks you ought to just let nature take its course and God will take care of you." She disagrees with this fatalistic attitude of an older generation, uses contraception.)

273. Girls are easier to raise than boys, cause they obeys you better, and they is closer to you when they grows up. (23T, 25T)

274. Seven girls . . . that's a whole lot of heads to comb! (46T, who had eleven children altogether, had "hoped for a boy to even things up.")

275. Boys are less trouble than girls. (46T, 9T, who had her first son after six girls, 17T, a very cleanliness-conscious ex-nurse.)

276. It's not that I don't trust my boyfriend around my kids--I do, but I have to think hard about bringing a man that's not their own father to actually live in the house. you know. (46T, whose last three children were by one man, and who was "thinking about getting married, maybe within the year." She had eleven illegitimate children, two of them teenage daughters, and expressed much anxiety to protect them from a fate similar to hers.)

277. I'm there all the time, and it's "Mommy this, and Mommy that." That's how I raises them, so they's all spoilt. (50T, who said that the neighbor now caring for her seven at home "don't see how anybody with all them kids could spoil every one of them that way!" This was more a boast than a complaint, however.)

278. We gonna buy everything new for this one because it'll be the last. We're intending to spoil this one good an proper! (50T, who had a tubal ligation after this, her eighth child.)

279. Whether you lives in a slum, or either in one of them rich sections, it don't matter--as long as you keeps yourself and your children clean, then you're a little bit special. Whereas even if you're rich, you might let your children run in the street all dirty. (13T, who took pride in working hard at her housekeeping, even though she suffered from a heart condition, and wasn't supposed to.)

280. People don't have no shame like they used to. You sees them sitting on the front steps nursing they babies--and sometimes they do it even in the Acme or on the bus! (42T, who was one of the mothers who rather expressed revulsion at nursing generally. Objectively speaking this cannot be commonly true--since so few mothers breast feed.)

281. I went to the doctor, and he told me I was pregnant. I was really scared, you know? Then I told my mother, and she said "why, that's nice!" and I stopped being so scared. (48T, who had fractured her pelvis in an auto accident at age 16 and been told that she might never be able to bear children as a result. Here is an obvious exception to the initiation of young women through scare stories, since reassurance was immediately given the young woman by her mother. Birth was normal, so evidently the doctor's scare story was unwarranted in her case.)

282. Until the birth certificate is made out, the baby has no name. (22T. This curious reliance on documents to make real the naming of one's child was quite common. Picking out a name was not enough--it had to be on the birth certificate before it was final. Until then women often changed their minds three or four times about the name, and they appeared rather relieved when the matter was out of their hands at last. Spelling of names was often a problem, too, and the sometimes-bizarre spellings women chose were frequently garbled by the clerk in charge of birth certificates. Women usually insisted that these be changed, and they were.)

283. The dead come back sometimes. (26T, and 15T, both tellers of tales.)

284. People say sometimes dead people's spirits can come back to bother the living. (14P, 13T)

285. My mother-in-law, she knows how to work them roots. She can put spells on people to drive them crazy. (13T, who says she hasn't eaten a meal in the mother-in-law's house since learning of her "root-doctoring" because she's afraid she'll "root something I eats." 9T also spoke of root-doctoring and of "witches who puts curses on people to drive them crazy, down in the backwoods in the South. Nobody won't tell you that's what they do, though, because it's against the law. But I seen it done.")[11]

FOOTNOTES--CHAPTER VI

[1]Newman (1965:126) rejects the use of the term "superstition" in favor of "beliefs" on grounds that "1) the term superstition is prejudicial, 2) some of the beliefs listed are patently true, and 3) an interesting aspect of the beliefs is the extension of the traditional form to include 'rational' or 'medically proven' content."

If it is true, as Levi-Strauss maintains (1966:Chapter 1) that magic and science spring from the same universal human "thirst for objective knowledge" and the equally universal human need to order such knowledge, the distinction between 'medically proven' or 'rational' belief and superstition is not the crucial one in the present context. The real distinction, as Levi-Strauss points out, is not that magic is less rational than science, but that it is more deterministic--it seeks certainty where science does not. Thus it can be noted in the present context, for example, that "superstition" seeks determinism in realms such as the prediction of the sex of infants, where science still hesitates to venture for lack of evidence. Similarly, superstition seeks to account for the occurrence of major or minor imperfections in infants through prenatal influence, where science has little to say. One can observe, however, the tendency for "better" (i.e., more scientific) explanations to supplant the traditional beliefs where these are available to the informants. One can attribute this, perhaps, to the simple diffusion downward in the social structure of the belief system of an elite--but this does not explain the process, it only describes it. If, however, there is an innate tendency in human beings to make the "universe an object of thought" and to order it rationally, the tendency for magical beliefs to be supplanted by more demonstrably rational ones is explained.

If, then, superstitious or magical beliefs stem from precisely the same innate tendency of the human mind as do scientific ones, magical systems exist, in some sense, at the same level as do scientific ones. It therefore seems unnecessary to discard the term itself as pejorative--and I will, therefore, use it interchangeably with the term "belief."

[2]Thus, in the example given above, the <u>structure</u> of both beliefs is identical (and of the form "if A, then B"). The difference which classifies winter babies' fate in the category of "signs" and the effect on the child of its mother's "evil" disposition as part of "magic" lies in the nature of the agents (the first non-human and impersonal, the second human and active). The agent's nature, of course, belongs to the <u>content</u> of the beliefs, not their structure.

[3]Spiro (1966) defines man's basic needs as falling under three major headings: the cognitive, the substantive, and the expressive. All three of these may be seen as being served by the transmission of folk beliefs, always with the Spirovian proviso that other forms of knowledge of greater functional utility are absent in the group being investigated.

[4]"Fict" is a term used by Honko (1968:13) to denote a class of items which are never really believed by adults, but are sometimes used to control or answer the embarrassing questions of small children. "Boogeyman" stories, "stork" stories, and

similar items fall in this category.

[5]Of interest here is the fact that an African Negro woman, who is not part of my sample, but with whom I spent some time when she was hospitalized for prenatal complications, reported that she found many of the same beliefs about prediction of sex among her ghetto neighbors as were current in her village in South Africa. I do not know, of course, whether these are beliefs which Bantu peoples caught from the Boers, or vice versa--the similarities had mainly to do with predicting sex from the manner in which the mother carries (high, low, round, pointed, etc.).

[6]This comes from two sources--a teacher at Gratz High School, and an ex-counsellor at Germantown High School. Both schools are nearly all black.

[7]This is not, of course, confined to American Negro culture. In Thailand, for example, it is believed that the first three days of life are precarious ones, for the baby still belongs to the spirits, who may take his soul unless one takes precautions to deceive them into thinking the baby is ugly and worthless. European "evil eye" beliefs emphasize the vulnerability of small babies to having their souls captured by some supernatural agency. Wordworth's "trailing clouds of glory" emphasized the closeness of the infant's soul to it's birthplace in heaven. The illustrations of this kind of belief are nearly endless.

[8]Signor, who reports in a newspaper article upon the first systematic research ever done upon this phenomenon. The article is based upon the work of Dubach, Brown, and Minnich, and one of the statements in it calls attention to the prevalence of pica among black women in the United States.

[9]I do not have documentation on this research, which I understand is now in progress at Lankenau Hospital, and has not reached the stage of publication. The research grew out of school performance of a group of lower-class Negro children in a Get-Set program, when their poor attention span and general lassitude prompted teachers to instigate physical checkups for a whole group of 3 and 4 year olds. When a very great number of the children were found to be quite anemic they were given iron orally, but failed to respond. Subsequently they did respond to iron injections. The mechanism which prevented absorption of iron from food and "tonics" in these children is not understood, but their mothers all had pica, and reported having it during pregnancy.

[10]Private conversation with Hope Thompson, Director of Social Services at TUH. Her observation is borne out by my own observations on the ward. The youngest mothers, if their babies were premature, were generally rather unconcerned about it, whereas older women usually were quite anxious about the baby's welfare. One girl of fourteen who miscarried after a long and serious illness remarked, when I expressed sympathy, "I don't care. I didn't need it, anyway." This girl was not one of my informants, since she was too ill to be interviewed during most of her hospital stay.

[11]Closely connected with root-doctoring and witchcraft is the giving of "readings" by women supposed to be gifted in seeing the future. Unlike the gypsy readings,

this is done without tea leaves or crystal ball, merely by "looking in a person's eyes," where the future can be read. One highly educated black social worker in the hospital freely admitted to an irrational fear of "being read"--a hangover from her childhood in a family where occult powers were believed in. When a patient offered her a free "reading" in gratitude for help given, "I ran out of there! Nobody's going to read me!" Judging from her response, I would say that my own estimates of the degree of belief in occult practices and ideas throughout this thesis may err on the side of conservatism, if anything. That is, I have more likely underestimated than overestimated the adherence to occult notions--possibly because I lack such faith myself.

CHAPTER VII

DISCUSSION AND CONCLUSIONS

As Paul Radin once remarked, every man is at once the creature, the creator, the carrier and the manipulator of his culture. Perhaps it is for this reason that it sometimes seems to the investigator that the cultural picture which may be inferred from behavior--either verbal or non-verbal--is one characterized more by diversity than by uniformity. In the present instance, for example, it often seemed to me that the differences between the cultural symbols and rules expressed among my informants, even through the stereotyped form of communication represented by the folklore, were more striking than the similarities. Thus when taken in the context of an individual's life experience an item of belief often conveyed quite different perceptions of the world, quite different meaning, than the same item found in the context of another life.

This impression of diversity becomes most vivid, perhaps, when one attempts the investigation of groups within complex and heterogeneous civilizations such as our own. Some such phenomenon is probably at the root of the proposition put forth by some theorists that culture is not received holistically at all, even though this assumption has underlain much traditional anthropological analysis (Cf. Kluckhohn, 1958; Wallace, 1961; and Douglas, 1966). An analogy may perhaps be drawn, with some justification, to the learning of speech. Just as each person may be said to speak an idiolect of his native language, so may each be said to hold his own peculiar version of his native culture. Thus, although like speech culture is acquired because of the innate capacity of human beings for learning it, it will (again like speech) be conditioned in its precise formulation and expression by many individual and situational factors.

It is by now a truism that it is neither necessary nor, perhaps, functionally useful for all individuals to share identical world views, values and norms in order for societies to maintain their integrity and order. In place of this simplistic older assumption, theorists have instead stressed the significance of the range of variation, both cultural and behavioral, within a society (Geertz, 1959) as well as the need for complementarity of roles, functions, and their cultural supports within any given society (Wallace, 1961).

Following this line of reasoning, it may be most useful to think of a "whole culture" as a kind of reservoir from which each person may dip that portion of the common store of cultural ideas which is best suited to his own status and roles within the society, and those most nearly compatible with his own needs, situation and personality. Thus, rather than each of us carrying a unique culture, each of us is the possessor of a partial culture, for even in the very simplest groups no single individual is in possession of all the ideas his culture has ever generated. The fact that these partial or personal versions of culture are dipped from the reservoir belonging to the society as a whole permits that congruence between individual versions which enables people to live and work in concert to maintain the social system.

It is the areas of overlap that I must deal with here in order to give a coherent account of what may be learned from the corpus of folklore already presented. However it is a wise idea, perhaps, to indicate at least briefly the wide differences in what I call "personal culture" which may exist between women whose sociological characteristics are almost identical. I have, therefore, selected three of my informants, all unmarried, all twenty years of age or younger, all Philadelphia-born, all having their first or second child, and all DPA recipients at the time they first registered in clinic. (One, whose "common-law husband" had taken a very low-paying job one month before her baby's birth was no longer a recipient at the time I interviewed her, however.)

The point of this exercise is to introduce a note of caution into the reader's view of the generalizations which will follow, and to promote an awareness in both reader and writer that the phenomenon dealt with--the subculture of the black ghetto--is by no means simple or uniform in its influence and that, furthermore, it interacts continually with "mainstream" culture. These cases are also a demonstration of the assertions made above, concerning the way in which culture may be differentially ingested and expressed by different individuals.

Case 1.

Margaret was a fifteen year old girl who had just given birth to a healthy boy after a labor which she described as neither very prolonged nor very "bad." She considered herself lucky that she had needed no "stitches" following delivery, and was rather elated that she was therefore suffering none of the postpartum discomforts which were being experienced by her neighbor in the next bed. She agreed with this neighbor that she must be "stronger" than some other girls, and smiled over this fact. She also connected her own childbearing capabilities with those of her mother, who had a tubal ligation at the age of thirty-seven after bearing twins, her eleventh and twelfth live births. Even this event, said Margaret, had not been due to a decline in her mother's ability to bear children. It was simply that "she didn't want any more. But the doctors told her she was still good enough to have as many more as she already got!"

Margaret was now the eldest surviving of her widowed mother's twelve children. An older sister, aged seventeen, had died about a year earlier following the birth of her first child--a fact which seemingly accounted for Margaret's report of her own extreme nervousness during pregnancy. She described herself as having exhibited a change in personality, in fact, so that she lost interest in music, dancing and social life, and often suffered attacks of "shakes" during which she often rocked back and forth until her mother predicted that "the baby would rock after it was born."

Margaret's mother had several pre-school children of her own, as well as her orphaned grandchild to take care of, and it seemed certain that she would be in charge of rearing Margaret's baby as well. Margaret saw herself rather in the role of helpful daughter than as a mother in her own right. She did not, however, plan to return to junior high school, but expected to stay home to "help out with all the children, since she hadn't liked school anyway.

It was not certain that Margaret knew of the connection between intercourse and pregnancy at the time she herself became pregnant, nor would she discuss the putative father of her child. His name didn't appear in the hospital records, either, causing me to suspect that she either had been abandoned by him or didn't know for sure who he was--for she was quite communicative on other topics. She knew, for example, numerous signs of pregnancy, all of which she remembered experiencing, but some of which she considered to be universal as against others which were peculiar to her own experiences. The universal signs were: cessation of the menses, swelling of the breasts, abnormal hunger, fainting spells and "getting fat." All of these she had observed not only in herself but in a school friend who became pregnant at the same time she did. Less normal symptoms were swelling of her hands and feet and excessive weight gain. Special diet precautions were necessitated by the latter symptoms, but although Margaret's anxious mother attempted to carry these out Margaret used to "cheat" whenever she had the chance. Margaret reported that her mother was so worried about her, due to the recent death of the eldest daughter, that she skipped her customary church attendance during the period of Margaret's pregnancy so as to leave her alone as little as possible.

Margaret was a small fount of information about folk methods of producing abortion, citing pepper drunk in hot water, castor oil taken in hot water and sitzbaths with mustard in them, taken as hot as one could bear. She herself, however, had been afraid to try any of these things, for she remembered that her mother had produced abortions several times by such means, and that on one occasion she had nearly bled to death as a result. A neighbor girl, too, had become very ill following a homemade abortion. She hinted, however, that she had tried other, more "innocent" means to get rid of the unborn baby. She believed that raising one's arms above one's head might cause the baby to be strangled by the umbilical cord, and that pushing heavy furniture might cause miscarriage, and reported that she had hung a lot of clothes and "cleaned house a lot" when she was pregnant.

Both Margaret and her mother, whom I later met, had "known" the baby would be a boy, because she carried high. Her mother also believed in and followed the custom of putting a dime in the new baby's hand to bring it luck. The mother's beliefs are not relevant here except in that they were transmitted to Margaret, but she might be mentioned here as one of the women who insisted that she could tell certain things long before the doctors were able to detect them. She cited the fact that she had known her last birth would be twins, because her legs had felt sore early in her pregnancy.

Margaret was an amiable girl, rather slow of speech and appearing somewhat dull. It is clear, however, that she was able to produce material from the general store of folklore which demonstrated a knowledge of non-occult signs serving as predictors of pregnancy, a well-developed notion of the validation of femininity through childbearing, and a concept of "strength" closely connected with the capacity to have children and to bear them easily. In addition there was an implicit belief in the moral and physical danger of deliberately aborting--although the moral danger was less compelling than the fear of death. Her own dependency on her mother for help and care was strongly emphasized--Margaret, though now a mother herself, was not yet ready to fully assume the adult or the nurturing role, and emphasized her status as daughter. It was left to her mother to function as the nurturing head of the family, both during Margaret's pregnancy and after her child's birth.

Case 2.

Carolyn was twenty years old, and had just given birth to her second son when I met her. Her first child was one year of age when the second was born, and until a month before this baby's birth Carolyn had received public assistance for most of the past year. Although this young woman was officially unmarried and retained her maiden name, she considered herself to be living in "common-law" marriage with the father of her two children, and in fact resided with him in his mother's household, and referred to her "husband" and her "mother-in-law" during interviews. Her own parents were reported as being stable working class people who have lived for thirty years in the same home in Germantown. They had disapproved strongly of Carolyn's dropping out of high school shortly before graduation because she was pregnant, and of her going to live in "common-law" marriage with her present "husband." They became reconciled, however, after the first child's birth, and despite disapproval of Carolyn's irregular marital status took an interest in her and the children, perhaps because Carolyn was their only child. Carolyn's mother, in fact, was the source of many of the numerous home remedies which this bright, lively girl produced.

Carolyn believed that dreams could predict the future, and said that her mother-in-law was gifted with a capacity to do this. She had known "before I knew it myself" on both occasions when Carolyn became pregnant, and had known "by having a dream"--but Carolyn didn't know what sort of dream it had been. Her own first certain knowledge of her pregnancies came when she began to miss her menstrual periods.

The sex of unborn children, this young woman believed, could be predicted. If a woman carries high, she'll have a boy, and if she carries low, a girl. The "signs" didn't apply in her own case this second time, however, because Carolyn found herself carrying lopsided--and speculated that carrying her other baby around on one hip all the time had been the cause of this. ("Something I had no business doing," she added, since excessive strain in pregnancy is supposed to be bad for you.) Carolyn had also heard that one could predict the sex of babies by the way the mother's hair grew during pregnancy, and that "if it's a boy, the mother's hair will grow long, and if it's a girl her hair will fall out." She traced beliefs of this variety to their origins in the South, even though both she and her mother were born in Philadelphia. Her grandmother had been born in Virginia, she said, and still held to many "old-time" beliefs, which she transmitted to her daughter and granddaughter.

Carolyn herself believed quite openly in explanations which were occult or which she knew quite well to be at variance with scientific explanations and predictions. Her own child, for example, had been born just when a neighbor had told her it would be--at the moon's change of phase, the night after full moon. Furthermore, her husband had suffered low back pains throughout her labors with both this and her other child. This was because she had followed her grandmother's advice to crawl over her husband three times in bed during her pregnancy, thus inducing her own symptoms in him. He had also suffered from unusual hunger while she was pregnant, and had grown quite fat as a result.

A mother, Carolyn believed firmly, knew better than any doctor when her baby was "ready to be born." She could not describe precisely how she knew, but described it as a feeling "like a instinct" which had told her both times that delivery was imminent, even though both her children had been a bit early in coming.

Carolyn hadn't told her mother or grandmother immediately when she became pregnant. Even so, her grandmother had known "before my belly showed at all yet, by looking in my eyes. She said "they looked all clear and shiny, and that's how you can tell a girl is pregnant." During pregnancy, too, a woman's skin becomes clearer, and her nails grow faster than usual.

Prenatal influences can definitely mark the baby, Carolyn told me. Her own mother had marked her, she said, with a pinkish mark that resembled "the heart of a watermelon" which was caused by her mother's unsatisfied craving for that fruit during her pregnancy. Carolyn knew of numerous other examples in which prenatal cravings, left unsatisfied, had led to marking. She also knew that one should be careful never to laugh at a handicapped person during pregnancy, "or else your child will be born looking like that person." She also more than half-believed that laughing at a friend who is pregnant will soon cause one to become pregnant oneself--in fact she remembered razzing a friend of hers just about nine months before the birth of her second baby. The friend had warned her that she'd soon be pregnant herself, and sure enough "my first baby is only a year old, and here I am."

At the time Carolyn was confined the scandal of the ward was the case of a seventeen year old girl who was giving her baby up for adoption. This phenomenon was viewed by Carolyn, as well as many other women, as utterly unnatural. She couldn't imagine how a woman could "carry a child for nine months and then give it away to someone else." She herself had been offered a chance to give her first baby away to a childless middle-aged couple, but had refused, and felt that with public assistance available, even a mother who was "all alone in the world" (as she herself was not) could manage to keep her baby with her, or at least retain the right to see it.

Carolyn had many remedies for minor ailments of early infancy, most of them from her mother and grandmother. She had great respect, in particular, for her mother's medical know-how, saying that she "ought to have been a doctor." Gum "asafizzity" made into an infusion and added to the baby's bottle is good for both colic and for fevers accompanying difficult teething. Some people hang the same substance, in root form, around the baby's neck on a string to "draw out the fever"--but Carolyn preferred her mother's recipe. "Sweet niter" is another remedy which can be given for fevers, mixed in a bit of sugar water. It is also good to rub on a baby's gums to relieve teething pain.

Carolyn knew precisely how conception takes place and had a scientific vocabulary for describing the process. Thus, although old-time remedies were considered sufficient for the treatment of minor maladies of infancy, the matter of preventing conception was quite another sort of thing, and she preferred to rely on the latest of modern medical techniques. Before she left the hospital, therefore, she requested that the doctor install a "coil"--and she knew that she must watch carefully and return at once to the hospital if it should be expelled.

For a girl barely twenty years old, Carolyn was unusual in both the amount and nature of the lore she possessed--the accumulated folk and medical wisdom of three generations of capable women, one gathered. The lore which Carolyn possessed reveals, first of all, her confidence that knowledge is possible and that it gives one the power to cope with the exigencies of having and rearing children. There are many ways to predict what will happen to you, and there are effective ways of dealing with events if you take an active role in helping yourself. Pregnancy was seen by Carolyn as an essentially benign state in which one's hair, skin and nails are likely to improve--perhaps a reflection of her own healthy pregnancy and a general sense of security in her husband's and family's love and concern (demonstrated in the former case by the husband's sympathetic symptoms). She also had a view of mother and child as autonomous, and as knowing, better than the doctors, what would take place and when. A mother's instinct, born of the mystical identity of mother and child, could be relied upon not only to see the pregnancy through successfully, but to keep her in the natural motherly relation to her child--that of caring for the child and keeping it with her. Bright, independent-minded and pragmatic in her general outlook, Carolyn was willing to accept any remedy or technique she felt to be well proven as working--and had no prejudices either for or against modern science, being just as willing to draw upon it for solutions as she was willing to draw on the fund of traditional knowledge. She was interested in those techniques which were least expensive and most effective, no matter where they came from.

This same independence and practicality may well have been the reason why Carolyn had kept her relationship with the father of her children extra-legal, even though she was fond of her husband, lived with his family, and the union was of some duration. She viewed her children as being primarily hers, and legal marriage might have jeopardized her total control of them at some future date, so that pragmatic factors dictated that things were perhaps best left as they presently were.

Case 3.

Shirley was a sixteen year old high school girl whom I first met during the sixth month of her pregnancy, when she was hospitalized for suspected "kidney trouble." She tended to discount the diagnosis because she was feeling fine, and she was annoyed at being in the hospital. Shirley said that she had been doing well in school before she became pregnant, and that she intended going back to finish high school after the birth of her baby. She intended leaving the infant in her mother's care, or with a babysitter, and attending both day and night classes so that she could catch up to her classmates in time to graduate with her original class.

Shirley lived with her mother and four siblings, two older sisters and two younger brothers. The nineteen year old sister who is the eldest at home had two children and was currently pregnant with a third. Shirley said that, in the past, she had often asked this sister questions about sex, but the sister would never answer her. Her mother never told her anything at all about having babies, and Shirley felt too embarrassed to ask her about the matter. Thus one gathered that despite being a fairly bright girl, Shirley had only scattered and inaccurate information about sex when she herself became pregnant. Although she was still embarrassed to talk about it, it seemed likely that she had known too little to avoid pregnancy for herself.

She had, however, known that a missed menstrual period might be a sign that she was pregnant. She also knew that one might take "the pill" to prevent conception, but her older sister had taken them and "they gave her a whole lot of clots on her stomach, and she had three periods in one month and gained forty-five pounds" so Shirley was afraid to take them. Instead she announced her intention of using the "coil" after the birth of this baby.

Shirley was rather shy, and volunteered little information of her own accord during the interview, at which two other patients were present. She had heard of several beliefs proffered by others, however, although she showed little disposition to believe them. She had heard that "if you have a lot of heartburn while you're pregnant the baby will have lots of hair," and also that wiping a baby's face with its own wet diaper will "make its skin pretty." She had also heard a variant of the belief that a girl child clinging to the mother during pregnancy will "mark it (the new baby) for a girl." Her own version came as a memorate about a friend's little sister, who "didn't like my friend the whole time she was pregnant. She wouldn't come near her, even though she always hung around her a lot before that. Everybody said her little sister was jealous because another little girl was coming." When the new baby turned out to be a girl after all, Shirley found herself half-convinced that the little sister's behavior had, somehow, been significant.

Shirley had undergone a hazing of a sort at the hands of her older sisters when it was discovered that she was pregnant. One had frightened her about the pelvic examinations, telling her that "the doctors would shove something up inside me, and that it would hurt--and it did, too." When the doctors had hazarded a guess that she might be bearing twins, her sisters teased her about needing two names for her babies. Shirley, thinking that one baby was already one too many, didn't appreciate the joke. She was personally hoping for a girl, although she didn't really believe that one could predict sex. (Two months later she actually did give birth to a little girl, and seemed rather pleased, despite her original dislike of having a baby.)

Shirley, displeased at her condition, annoyed at being in the hospital, and still thinking of herself as a schoolgirl rather than as a mother, was not a very fertile source of folklore. She seemed to reject too-deep involvement with the whole transition to adult status by wanting to know as little as possible about it. On the other hand, she did show interest in contraception, the means of avoiding similar situations in future. There was obvious resentment at her older sister's failure to inform her about sex in such a way that pregnancy might have been avoided, but interestingly enough she did not blame her mother for the same omission. After all, she hadn't asked her mother--and it was plain that she felt embarrassed at the thought of discussing intimate sexual matters with her, or even thought it improper.

Shirley made no mention of the father of her child, but did refer to her boyfriend's mother as being a friendly party. She intended, in fact (evidently as a diplomatic move intended to flatter her through conferring an honor upon her) to allow her to name the baby. The entire context of the discussion made it plain, in fact, that when it came to childbearing the significant persons to be relied upon were a female contingent composed of mother, sisters, and boyfriend's mother, and not the baby's father.

Even the fairly scant material produced by this informant shows certain definite concerns as ranking high in importance. Being pregnant at this time in her life was experienced as a misfortune, even a punishment, but since it was a punishment incurred through ignorance rather than intention it was resented. The sphere of knowledge in which she showed the most interest, therefore, was that which would enable her to avoid future mishaps of the same nature--i.e., contraception. The conception of male and female roles, too, came through rather clearly--with males bearing little or no responsibility for the females they impregnate. Rejection of the maternal role was, in Shirley's case, symbolized by her clinging to the schoolgirl role and taking little interest in matters concerned with the baby or its fate. Nevertheless, she was not contemplating giving the child up, and when it finally arrived showed some pleasure in it, in accordance with cultural expectations.

The three cases just cited serve as illustrations of the way in which three individuals who would look nearly indistinguishable on a chart specifying their sociological characteristics have absorbed quite different kinds and amounts of material from the cultural reservoir available to them. It requires extended case study, therefore (only briefly summarized here) to locate the possible factors responsible for their differential ingestion of such cultural values as are exemplified in the folklore. What is evident is that while there is overlap between the areas of concern they exhibit, there is very variable emphasis, and sometimes even contradiction in the cultural attitudes adopted and expressed by different individuals.

It is the areas of overlap, however, which are the concern of one attempting to determine the total contents of the reservoir -- or at least the contents of this particular pool, which centers around procreation.

I have earlier adopted a definition of folklore which states that it is a process of communication. Now I shall attempt to analyze what it is that is being communicated.

Abstracting Value Premises from the Folklore

For purposes of analysis I have surveyed the corpus of lore and arrived inductively at a series of contrast categories which are at that level of abstraction which Miller (1965) called "focal concerns," Kluckhohn (1958) called "value premises," and Redfield (1953:84) referred to as aspects of "world view." These high-level abstractions are associated with groups of lower level ones termed, most commonly, values --either positive or negative--and values in turn are determinants of those rules or expectations which are the cultural norms or directives (though sometimes not of the behavioral ones to be statistically discovered on the ground).

The contrastive categories are relative in nature, rather than absolute. That is, they are not Levi-Straussian oppositions, in need of mediation, but rather polar extremes of a series of continua within the cultural system. Most relevant values and norms will fall somewhere between them, therefore. Furthermore, being abstractions they are somewhat arbitrary and will be readily seen not to be mutually exclusive, but actually cross-cutting at many points. The list below does not, therefore, pretend to be exhaustive, or even the only possible list which might have been inferred from the materials at hand. It is merely a convenient and, I think, fruitful basis for discussion of the matter which is communicated by means of this particular body of folklore.

These are not "native categories of thought"--although I believe them to be implicitly present in "native minds" and recognizable by them as genuine areas of concern. The restricted nature of the situation to which they refer means, too, that the list doubtless fails to include categories which might emerge in some other context than the situation of childbearing, or among men rather than among women. Furthermore, some of the concerns listed here are more intimately and exclusively connected with procreation *per se* than are others, which may have much wider applications in the total sub-culture.[1] The list, then, with all these qualifications, follows:

1. Knowledge vs. ignorance
2. Fate vs. free-will
3. Autonomy vs. dependence

4. Strength vs. weakness
5. Then vs. now.
6. Rational vs. irrational
7. Normal vs. abnormal
8. Reward vs. punishment
9. Kin vs. non-kin
10. Maleness vs. femaleness
11. Nurturance vs. deprivation
12. Legitimate vs. illegitimate

These concerns are formulated at the abstract level of world-view, as had already been indicated, with values and norms viewed as being derivative of that "highest" level of abstraction. This statement, however, is a logical one, not a historical one. No one can determine whether the norms or directives actually give rise to an appropriate set of values or world-view, or vice versa, and therefore I make no conjectures about historical causality. In actuality there is undoubtedly a complex interaction going on between the conceptually "separate" levels of cultural abstraction, but the precise nature of this interaction is far too large a subject to be dealt with here, and may be inaccessible to empirical investigation. I shall, then, move on to discuss the categories in the terms already outlined--as major value premises, values and norms derived inferentially from the lore and the context of its expression.

1. Knowledge vs. ignorance

That "knowledge is power" is a truism of human existence. This knowledge can exist in several forms--as that necessary for predicting events, or as that necessary for understanding or controlling them. One could, in fact, defend the notion that the most important aspect of the world view of any culture has to do with what is and what is not a subject for human knowledge, and with the epistemological problem of how we know what we know.

In the view of my informants there is more than one way of knowing. The most reliable, or at any rate the most commonplace, is naturalistic in mode. Pregnancy is something that one can know about, and childbirth therefore something that one can predict from a basic knowledge of one's own biological "signs." (Thus belief #1 is very nearly universal.) There are alternative ways of knowing, however, that one is pregnant--and these smack of the occult, or at any rate of the non-physical universe. Thus emotional signs (Cf. #8 through 12) may signify pregnancy before it becomes obvious otherwise, with a woman becoming "evil" or spiteful. Or such mysterious occult signs as dreams may serve as means of knowing in advance of the physical symptoms' appearance (Cf #14 through 16).

The sex of the unborn, too, may be predicted by means of a variety of signs--so conveniently various and contradictory that one can nearly always, if one is so inclined, lay claim to having "known all the time." This is certainly enhancing to a woman's feeling of power, even though only one such belief refers even jocularly to any possible means by which one might actively influence the sex of the unborn child (Cf. #219). For the most part the power conferred by "knowledge" in this area is adjustive--that is, one may make one's peace with the inevitable possibility that one may not have the sort of baby one would like. Here, again, some of the signs are straightforward physical manifestations, such as the shape of one's belly, while others are more mysterious and subtle, such as the behavior of other children of the same sex who may "hang on" or avoid the pregnant woman (Cf. #18 through 28, #37 through 40).

Many direct causal relationships are subjects of knowledge, and these imply potential control. Biological knowledge concerning the manner in which one becomes pregnant and eventually delivers open the possibility of preventing conception, or even of aborting once pregnancy has occurred. Thus there is a whole complex of beliefs concerning contraception both by means of personal restraint (Cf. #62 and 63) and by means of medical intervention (Cf. #67, 72, 73, 74, 75) as well as many which involve knowing techniques for abortion (Cf. #177 through 187). Both contraception and abortion techniques, however, may carry negative as well as positive values, for they (and particularly the latter) can place a woman in physical danger (Cf. #178, 183, 158, 159) while abortion is a source of acute moral danger as well (Cf. #160).

The responsibility to impart knowledge about childbearing is thought to reside rightfully with one's mother--or perhaps an older sister. Thus, even though only three informants actually reported learning the "facts of life" from their own mothers prior to their first pregnancy, many were resentful of the negligence or inhibition which had left them thus vulnerable at a crucial time of their lives, and vowed that they would not similarly neglect the education of their own daughters.

Early sex education for most of my informants came from a "girlfriend" or "kids at school" and was, of course, often inaccurate. This usually occurred during the junior high school years, which is when a large number of girls had become pregnant the first time. (Thirteen of my fifty informants had given birth to their first child before the age of sixteen, and only one was married at that time. Some of the girls had later married the father of that first child, usually when they were pregnant by him once again.) Nearly all who discussed their very early pregnancies spoke of their shock, fear, and unreadiness for motherhood, and several described themselves as having become extremely nervous and upset during the first pregnancy.[2] There is, then, a great deal at stake where adolescent girls are suffered to live in ignorance of the consequences of sex, and such ignorance is valued very negatively among my informants, even though it may be statistically common.

It seems fair to state that much of the knowledge a woman has of the process of procreation is learned, in this group, at the cost of her own or a friend's difficult early experience of "getting caught," following an act she didn't really know could lead to pregnancy. Thus we have a paradox arising, in that girls who know a great deal about sex, and who may have known it well before they reached adolescence, often know nothing about its consequences until it is too late. The policy implications for educators are, of course, rather obvious. The standard sex education course given in eleventh or twelfth grade is scheduled far too late for ghetto girls, and probably for many others as well.

Nearly all the beliefs deal with knowledge of one sort or another, of course. There is knowledge of potential danger: a man should never beat a pregnant woman, for example (Cf. #141) nor should a woman have too many babies, in quick succession (Cf. #155). Trouble during one pregnancy presages possible trouble with subsequent ones, and therefore one should avoid these for the sake of both mother and child (Cf. #154). It is bad to eat starch, to get too fat, or to become too nervous--for these are seen as organic things affecting the unborn child as well as the mother (Cf. #117, 118, 127).

Just as positive knowledge is valued as a way of coping with the events connected with procreation, and ignorance of sex is seen as a handicap to one's ability to cope with its consequences, so too knowledge of the proper manner of bringing children up is positively valued. The lack of it is likely to result in a child's illness or death, or at the very least in his becoming spoiled. The doctor is viewed as the ultimate authority in the physical sphere, but where a woman considers that she already knows what is necessary she will seldom ask for medical advice or explanations. Unless, therefore, such advice is routinely offered and explained as it pertains to the individual case, women will go on doing things they "know" to be harmless (such as eating what they please, sometimes including starch) (Cf. #188 and 191 through 194).

In summary, then, knowledge of many sorts is seen as an important source of power and control for the individual. Knowledge may stem, however, from a variety of sources, natural and occult, internal and external, modern and traditional. There seems to be no distinct hierarchy of value regarding the way in which knowledge is attained, save that the person or other source transmitting it seem to be authoritative, and that the knowledge should be validated by testimony to the effect that it works. The standard is pragmatic, and the frame of reference personal and experiential rather than logical or abstract. Thus if a woman's experience convinces her that dreams are an even better (or at least earlier) sign of pregnancy than physiological signs she will accept such incompletely understood sources of knowledge as being quite as valid as those whose workings she may understand better. In this respect she may be very little different from most other Americans--or perhaps from most other human beings. Since, however, the knowledge provided by science tends on the whole to be more useful than that available through other modes of cognition there seems to be a general tendency for scientific knowledge, where it is available to my informants, to drive out less successful means of prediction, explanation and control. There are, however, many areas of concern in which science provides no ready answers. Since any sort of knowledge is more satisfying to individuals than is the acceptance of anomaly or ambiguity, the topics on which science remains silent are subjects for explanation by alternative means.

2. Fate vs. free will

Under this rubric are subsumed the mysterious forces over which man has no real control, as opposed to those over which he does have control. Both luck and fate are versions of the former orientation, and they are often the only explanations people can find for undeserved suffering, of which there is a great deal in the ghetto as elsewhere. Fate may wear a religious guise--the will of God--or it may be secularized as bad luck or good luck. In any case it is invoked to deal with the problem of suffering, which Weber pointed to as a central one for all human existence.

To the degree to which human beings are at the mercy of their fate they are powerless. To the degree to which they conceive of themselves as having free will and control over the courses of their lives, they possess power. Since my informants belong to a stratum of society which wields very little real material power, it is not surprising that many kinds of ill fortune are viewed as the unavoidable effects of powers beyond one's control. Still, fate is neither always malign nor always unavoidable. One may have good luck as well as bad, and one may practice numerous avoidances if one is determined to outwit fate. In the folklore are many prescriptions for avoidance which, if conscientiously followed, enable a woman to insure that her unborn child will be healthy and unblemished (Cf. beliefs on "marking" #100 through 116). In this area there is a conscious decision made through the exercise of one's own free will as to whether or not the observance of many taboos is worth the trouble. Frequently it is not--but few of the events seen as influential are truly unavoidable (Cf. two exceptions in #108 and 109). (Also, since one cannot always decide what time of year the baby will be born, #102 and 103 are relatively--though not seriously --"fateful".)

Luck is a concept closely related to fate, but perhaps more hopeful in its overtones, since it is as likely to be good as bad. This is closely connected, too, with a notion of personal freedom--one can calculate the odds, to a degree, and gamble on the outcome. Thus one may gamble on delaying the trip to the hospital while in labor, in order to avoid the discomfort and indignity of "them doctors messing you around," and if one is "lucky" one will manage to get to the hospital in time to be delivered safely and hygienically (Cf. #198). One can also attempt to influence luck, which is seen on occasion as a power that can be bribed with gifts or good works. Thus one places a dime in the new baby's hand to bring it luck in life, or one takes in an orphaned child to bring luck in the house. (Cf. #215, 68). On the other hand one shouldn't get too arrogant and presume that all will go well, and that one's baby will be born alive. For this reason one might hesitate to buy the infant's clothes before it is born (Cf. #136), for this amounts to tempting fate and may bring bad luck.

The relative lack of positive means for insuring the health, beauty and good fortune of one's unborn child is probably a reflection of empirical reality rather than of deep fatalism. It is certainly not a reflection of lack of maternal concern, for once a child is here, if it suffers some illness or defect the measures taken are active ones (Cf. #217, as well as the wide variety of cures: #232 through 254). Only one positive prenatal action--eating fish so that the baby would be "smart"--is recommended, in contrast to the host of suggested avoidances. There is perhaps, less of an obsessive insistence in the ghetto than there is elsewhere in U. S. society that every child be perfect, but whether this can be classed as fatalism or only as healthy realism is a matter of one's point of view.

3. Autonomy vs. Dependence

This category deals, essentially, with the self-concepts of my informants. It is closely related, of course, to their notions about fate. If fate is all powerful and all pervasive one cannot be autonomous--it is useless to take positive action of any sort. If, however, fate operates in a more limited way, if there are, indeed, areas of free will within which the individual can take action, one is not totally dependent on forces outside oneself.

Objectively speaking, the group of women under discussion is one which finds itself very restricted in some of the areas of autonomy and independence upon which the larger society places greatest value. Prime among these is economic independence. More than half of my informants are forced to live on public assistance, a particularly humiliating form of dependency which robs one of autonomy in many spheres of one's life.[3]

Childbearing is an important source of autonomy--one might almost say creativity--for ghetto women, who may feel inferior and powerless in so many other spheres. When it comes to having babies there are indications that my informants feel themselves to be a good deal more in control of the situation than do women in other segments of U. S. society (Cf. pp. 118-119). Thus although hospital care is decidedly the norm, and is certainly considered safest and most comfortable for the baby and the mother, it is not indispensible. Many women spoke of mothers and grandmothers who gave birth without medical assistance, and even without a midwife, and two had had their first one or two children delivered at home by midwives in different parts of the South (Cf. p. 67).

Since it is not thought to be impossible or necessarily catastrophic to give birth at home women often elect, as has been mentioned earlier, to stay at home during most of their labor. Here they can sit up or walk about, without being subject to the restraints imposed by being put in a hospital bed and ordered to remain there. At least five women asserted that this made them much more comfortable, and preferred the freedom from interference by doctors and nurses until as late in the course of labor as possible. These women wanted the doctor to deliver them, allright, but they themselves were the authorities on when the baby was due to come, and they themselves with their babies carried out the most important part of the entire enterprise (Cf. p. 41). This stands in marked contrast, I believe, to the standard middle-class American conception of birth, in which the doctor and the mother are active participants, and the baby merely a passive object of their efforts--with voluntary action reserved mainly to the doctor. Among my informants it is believed that the child has a will of its own, and that the mother, because she is so closely attuned to the life within her, may interpret this will and thus "know . . . even if it's not supposed to be time yet" when the baby will come. "I knew every time," said one mother of three children, "even the one that didn't live" (Cf. #122).

Autonomy in the sphere of preventing conception is rather new to ghetto people, since such knowledge has not been widely disseminated until recent changes in the law permitted the establishment of educational programs in the hospital and elsewhere. Of course, once women come to the hospital, they are already pregnant--so that the in-hospital program is somewhat like closing the barn door after the horse is gone. Nevertheless, such information is valued very positively, at least at a verbal level--for it opens the prospect of autonomous decision-making in a sphere which was once a matter of "fate" entirely, unless a woman chose to live in celibacy. Certainly contraception is being accepted to the degree that most women take a lively interest in its possibilities, and are taking contraceptive devices and prescriptions home with them. On the other hand, few women report that the present baby is one that they deliberately "planned"--only two, in fact, indicated that they had stopped using contraception deliberately in order to have a baby. Most pregnancies, therefore, were reported as "accidents"--though there is a strong presumption in my mind that these were not always real accidents, but in fact resulted from an unconscious wish for a child. Perhaps many such "accidents" are the consequence of a value conflict. Childbearing is, among these as among most of the world's women, the supreme validation of femininity, and nearly all desire children. The same conflict of values may, too, be an important reason for the ubiquity of beliefs about the possible bad side-effects of contraceptive measures. "The Pill" and the IUD, which are the most effective measures in general use are also those whose dangers are pointed up in the folklore, despite the fact that hospital lecture-films play down such dangers and the women are told that ill effects are rare (Cf. #72, 76, and 77 through 83). Thus, although it is seen as a good thing for a woman to have children only when she wishes them, and to limit her family to a size she can manage, there are decided discrepancies between this value and the behavioral norms based upon conflicting values and beliefs.

Abortion, of course, is a desperate expedient resorted to only <u>in extremis</u>. Since it is thought to be both dangerous and morally culpable ("when you really think about it, that's murder" said one informant) this is an act which is very negatively valued, even though it implies perhaps the ultimate autonomy on the part of the mother (Cf. #158, 159, 178, 271). It is better to submit to the will of God, or to one's bad luck and "go ahead and have it." Thus even though the nature of the evidence is such that one is convinced that many of the informants have entertained the notion of deliberate abortion, public opinion condemns it and women known to have tried it are subject to malicious gossip. Of course since all of my informants are members of that segment of the ghetto population who have carried the pregnancy through rather than endanger themselves and the child either physically or morally there is no way to judge how representative they may be of the female ghetto population <u>in toto</u>.

Tubal ligation is not similarly harshly judged, but is seen as a last resort of those who feel they cannot possibly face another pregnancy. This choice is not always a function of the absolute number of children a woman has borne, although there seems to be some reluctance on the part of physicians to perform such surgery on women under thirty or those whose families are relatively small. One woman, however, who had responsibility for eight children, even though only three were her own, decided that enough was enough and a tubal ligation was performed. Three others who were indeed worn out from childbearing were also operated on, and another who was severely diabetic had a tubal ligation for reasons of her own health after the birth of her second baby. Only one of these women had a legal husband (from whom she was separated) whose consent had to be obtained for the operation. Several other women who either had husbands living with them, or were separated but not on friendly terms with their legal mates wished for tubal ligations, but could not obtain the necessary consent. The decision to resort to tubal ligation may be seen as an autonomous act, but since it is one which permanently removes further autonomy in the sphere of procreation it occupies a somewhat anomalous position in the scale of values.

Much lip service is given to female dependence on medical advice and assistance during pregnancy and labor. Nevertheless it would seem that in reality it is at least equally important to follow one's own desires and instincts during pregnancy. The numerous beliefs endorsing self-indulgence of all kinds are indicative of the degree to which the women value behavioral latitude during pregnancy, and are reluctant to give it up. Thus "marking" beliefs frequently symbolize the importance of letting mothers eat as they please, and even those who have been told that such habits as starch-eating are "bad" are likely to indulge the habit (Cf. #85, 86, 91, 92).

In summary, then, the women of the ward are likely to feel that their autonomy, even in defiance of doctors' orders, is considerable in the sphere of childbearing. Their concept of the unborn child, too, is colored by the belief that a baby knows what it wants and should not be interfered with or manipulated (Cf. #122).

The belief in the child's autonomy is radically altered, however, once it is actually born. It is then the mother who decides things, not the child, who is conceived of as utterly dependent, and whose will is not important. When and how much clothing or other equipment is appropriate is for the adult to decide. (Cf. #225) Furthermore, a baby's demands for attention, unless they are interpreted as hunger, pain or illness, are not to be acceded to, for this will only "spoil" the child. Thus it is bad to hold a baby too much, or to rock it to sleep, for the more a baby is allowed to influence others by its demands the more likely it is to be difficult to control later on (Cf. #148, 149, 277). Maternal control over children is an important value, therefore "spoiling" is much frowned upon.[4]

Furthermore, the techniques for manipulating children are not subject to too many scrupulous considerations of honesty. Lying to children is routine, and is routine, and is rationalized by reference to the child's unreadiness for certain facts of life. This accounts for the variety of "ficts" used to fend off questions asked by older children about sex (Cf. #255 through 260). It is also permissible to promise things one has no intention of giving in order to manipulate children who, after all, have no real recourse or autonomy since they are dependent on the mother for everything.

The avoidances which have been mentioned earlier as examples of the attitude toward fate versus free-will may be viewed also as having a bearing on one's autonomy, since the categories are so closely related. Here it is only a kind of negative autonomy which is exercised, and the prohibitions and avoidances with which the folklore abounds are seldom or never observed in toto. There seems to be, rather, a selection of those avoidances which a woman deems as seriously important and therefore worth the effort of self control involved. What seems worth the trouble will be, of course, a function in part of the strength of the woman's belief, and in part of the sort of personality she is--whether easy-going and ready to trust to luck, or anxious and conscientious.

4. Strength vs. weakness

Power and strength are not synonymous, since power may also reside in one's knowledge or cleverness, or in one's intrinsic human autonomy. Nevertheless, strength is an important component of power, and in the ghetto it would seem that a woman's strength is measured to an important degree by her capacity to bear and rear children. These measures of strength are, of course, tied importantly to the entire concept of the feminine role, therefore the lack of childbearing strength is threatening to one's whole self-evaluation as a female. The importance of this aspect of the female self may indeed be one reason why large families persist in the black subculture of the city. Perhaps this is also a vestige of the time when, in the rural South, large families were an economic asset, and appropriate values were developed to endorse them (Cf. p. 43. See also #272 as an indication of explicit rejection by one informant of the traditional values expressed by her grandmother). Even if a woman decides to exercise her personal autonomy by limiting her family, however, it is important that significant others should understand that her strength is not impaired (Cf. p. 43).

Babies, in contrast to adults, are thought of as weak and fragile, a concept entirely consonant with their dependency and lack of real autonomy. Even a baby's soul, it is hinted, is but weakly attached to its body, so that a mother's watchfulness is needed to keep the angels or the devil from stealing it away (Cf. #57, 58, 227). It is the strength of women that brings babies into the world, and it is their knowledge and strength that keeps them here. Ideally, then, a mother is a tower of strength and protectiveness throughout her child's life--the person one can count on no matter what happens.

5. Then vs. now

Cultural concepts of the ordering of time are a subject of great complexity which cannot be fully dealt with in the present context. Here the single time-referent which emerges as important is the one I have dubbed "then vs. now"--but which might have been more aptly called "old people vs. young people" in connection with this body of data. It was this linguistic usage which cropped up again and again in the course of field work--sometimes with the addendum "down home" or "down in the South" to indicate where the geographic locus of old-time ideas was.

In this context, the generations are separated through explicit reference to differences in their beliefs and values regarding childbirth. Time and again an informant would preface the repetition of a belief which she herself rejected with "The old people say . . . ." In this sense the old people are often viewed as ignorant, superstitious and old-fashioned, and some of their beliefs as out-of-date nonsense (Cf. #81, 116, 162, 188, 205).

On the other hand, respect for the wisdom of elders is quite prominent in many of the beliefs. There is much faith in some of the "old time" cures which mothers and grandmothers employed for infant complaints, even though they are explicitly recognized as being quite at variance with modern medical practice, which the women also have some knowledge of. A grandmother may send the annual supply of "spring tonic" from the South each year, or prescribe old-fashioned root or herb concoctions for babies, and since these are usually cheaper than the remedies prescribed by doctors they may well be tried first (Cf. #189, 226, 228, 232 through 254).

In sum, one's elders are thought of in somewhat contradictory terms, even by one and the same person, as being ignorant in some respects and wise in others. There is, perhaps, greater dependency on the wisdom of older women among ghetto dwellers than there is in the population outside the ghetto, when all is said and done --perhaps because minor illnesses are seldom brought to a doctor. Since such complaints as teething fevers and colds are generally self-limiting anyway, home remedies proposed by "the old people" receive credit for the baby's recovery, for cures are seldom thought of as spontaneous (Cf. #241 and 242 for especially picturesque examples).

Serious illness, however, is the province of doctors. So is childbirth itself, and to a lesser extent prenatal care, although women who feel well may delay clinic registration or fail to register at all for economic reasons. In the matter of contraception, too, the "old ways" are seen as conspicuous failures, and modern medical prescriptions are generally the accepted means (Cf. #164 through 176).

With respect to childbearing the "old days" are seen as a time when pregnancy and labor were fraught with pain and danger, and perhaps with tragedy (Cf. #157). The fortitude of the "old people down in the South" is admired, and their survival is thought of as a sign of strength, but there is no wish to emulate them. Two women in my sample who had given birth to their first children in the South with only midwives or relatives to assist them were emphatic in their view that it was a great deal better to give birth in the hospital (Cf. #201). Generally, then, although "now" is far from perfect it is conceived of as being rather better than "then".

6. <u>Rational vs. irrational</u>

Order must exist in a cultural universe, and if it is an order that is capable of human apprehension through intellectual means it can be thought of as a rational universe. The power to know, which has been discussed earlier, is closely related in the Western world-view to rationality. Although there is, in some of the interstices of Western thought as well as in many non-Western cultures, the possibility of "knowing" things through direct revelatory or mystical experience, my informants do not speak of such experience, save with reference to prophetic dreams.

My informants generally adhere to the dominantly rational mode of Western thought, in which every effect must have a cause. This is extensively demonstrated by the whole category of causes, even though many of the items may seem to the scientifically oriented observer to be grounded in irrationality. One may, of course, distinguish categories of causes, some of which are "modern and scientific" and others of which, being incapable of verification by empirical means are not. Nevertheless they are all "rational" in essence because they operate in a knowable, systematic fashion.

Material causes of events are those most subject to verification. Thus the cause of pregnancy lies in a physical union of man and woman, and the cause of unwanted pregnancy is generally attributed to failure to employ the preventive measures now known to be available, or some failure of the technique itself which is explainable in material terms (Cf. #61 through 65, 67, 72 through 74, 84). No one, for example, suggests prayer as a means of avoiding conception. Similarly, most illnesses are thought of as having material causes, and the remedies for them are of a material nature for the most part (Cf. #191 through 195, 207 through 212 and 232 through 240).

An intermediate position in the scale is occupied by emotional causes. There is a mind-body relationship in which one's feelings and one's health are interrelated. Pregnancy can cause evil or spiteful behavior, for example, and a woman's emotional state can influence her delivery adversely (Cf. #127). Because strong emotions of an unpleasant kind can cause the baby to be born imperfect, there is a relation between the mother's emotions and the child's welfare, too (Cf. #105, 107, 109). The dependence of the child on its mother's state of mind is, however, also a part of the whole attitude about the total dependency of babies--therefore this category cross cuts with our third category as well. In any case it becomes a value here that the mother be helped to remain serene and happy during pregnancy so that she will have a healthy baby following an easy delivery.

Material and emotional causes of events in pregnancy do not, however, exhaust the possibilities of causal relationship. There are causes which lie in the supernatural realm. These, of course, are not so easily verifiable as the more common and observable material or emotional ones. Nevertheless they are conceived of in many cases as real, and as operating in rational and predictable ways. This allows human beings to exercise a degree of control--if only the negative one of avoidance --but there are persons who have special knowledge of a positive sort as well. Thus some people know how to "work them roots" (Cf. #213).

The supernatural is thought of as malign in its influence upon pregnant women and young infants, and therefore it is generally feared. Even the angels may want to steal one's baby's soul away, albeit more seductively than the devil (Cf. #57, 58). Still, one may apprehend the signs of such dangers and move to counteract them in a "rational" fashion, even if prediction is dependent on dreams, for example. One may predict, too, that a given individual born with a caul or with "holes in his ears" will be able to "see things" of a mysterious and immaterial nature, even though there may be nothing one can otherwise do about it (Cf. #50, 51). Thus even the supernatural forces of the universe follow patterned and predictable behavior, and in this sense are part of a rational world, and serve to supplement the more common and less frightening material explanations of things. The supernatural, then, fills some of the gaps in knowledge where science and everyday common sense remain silent or inconclusive. It completes the rationally ordered universe of events.

7. Normal vs. abnormal

What is normal is usually but not invariably normative as well. What most of the items or events in a given universe of similar things display in the way of characteristics is therefore "normal" even if it is undesirable or unpleasant, like the pain of childbirth, or the discomforts of pregnancy.

The "normal" may not, therefore, always be positively valued, since in itself it may be discommoding. Because of its statistical commoness, however, a certain amount of normal discomfort must be accepted.

Rarer statistical events, however, such as infant death or deformity, carry much greater negative valences, and may even be blamed on the mother if they are thought to have been caused by her (Cf. #137, 138, 140, 143). These are "abnormal" events which must be assigned a specific cause. A similar situation obtains for the "abnormal" phenomenon of sterility (Cf. #69, 70, 71).

It is normal for a woman to display certain vagaries of behavior during pregnancy, and to be allowed more latitude than would be given her at other times. Thus she may indulge in asocial behavior (Cf. #9, 11, 12) or a degree of gluttony which is neatly sanctioned by the belief that failure to satisfy her cravings will mark the baby (Cf. #100, 101).

It is, above all, normal for a woman to be strongly attached to her child, and therefore, the most unnatural thing a mother can do is to give a baby up for adoption (Cf. #146). It is likewise normal for a woman's husband or mate to show sympathy and concern for the woman he has impregnated, for the welfare of his unborn child, and to show pride in paternity. A father may demonstrate all three of these normal emotions through manifesting symptoms similar to those of pregnancy (Cf. #197). By this means he simultaneously asserts his paternity, his sympathy with the pregnant woman and his willingness to take responsibility and even discomfort on behalf of the child (Cf. #132, 197). Mothers whose husbands or boyfriends displayed such behavior regarded it as unusual enough to remark upon, but really as an intensification of valued behavior and feelings rather than as anything abnormal. The intensity of their mates' participation in their crisis of childbearing was, of course, very positively valued by the women who were lucky enough to have this sort of evidence of love.

8. <u>Reward vs. punishment</u>

Wrongdoing is punishable in every culture--and in our society, even wrongdoing which no one but the sinner himself is aware of, for if society does not mete out retribution then God or one's own conscience will.

Thus for laughing unkindly at a cripple, the mother may be punished by having her own child born similarly afflicted (Cf. #114, 220). If, on the other hand, a woman neglects her child and is not punished by God, society in the form of "them cruelty people" will step in and take her child away (Cf. #145). This latter belief, though formally stated only once, is widespread in more implicit forms, so that it becomes evident that women know that their control or "ownership" of their own children is exercised only within limits, with punishment for bad behavior.

A serious moral crime is to destroy the unborn by means of abortion. Here retribution may take the form of death for the mother as well as her child, and therefore, is deeply feared--probably quite realistically, one might add, and on other than moral grounds (Cf. #158, 159, 178, 183). But even if the transgressor should survive she may be punished by becoming sterile (and therefore lonely in her later years) or through the souls of her dead babies persecuting her when later she lies on her deathbed (Cf. #71, 160).

Reward for right action is the other side of the coin of retribution. A woman who endures the discomforts and dangers of pregnancy is entitled to a degree of indulgence and protection, as has already been mentioned. She may also evidence signs of enhanced beauty and well-being, perhaps as nature's compensation for the loss of her figure (Cf. #2, 3, 8).

The most serious of transgressions against the moral and natural order is a mother's rejection of her child. Placing a baby for adoption is the ultimate symbol of this rejection, for legal adoption is irrevocable. It is very nearly equivalent to a person's severing one of her own limbs, for there is ample confirmation in the lore (especially in beliefs about marking) that mother and child are thought of as so closely identified that they are nearly part of one another. Lesser degrees of rejection are not so harshly judged, however, and in fact are sometimes seen as practical solutions to difficult conditions. Thus it is a commonplace of ghetto existence that children are placed in foster homes of one or another variety, or raised by their grandmothers while the mother lives and works elsewhere. This, however, since it is not irrevocable, since the mother may repossess her child at any time she wishes, and since the child knows its own mother is not greatly frowned upon. The crucial factor seems to be a legalistic one, therefore, in that the mother does not give up her rights to the child, and is not therefore guilty of abandonment, as when she places her child for adoption. The punishment meted out for so doing is severe censure within the family and neighborhood, as well as the probable suffering a mother undergoes through knowing that her child will grow up loving someone other than its natural mother. The love of children for their mother is one of life's great rewards, and it is an unhappy woman who relinquishes it permanently.

Pregnancy itself can be treated punitively in the ghetto. It is not usual for this to occur when the girl is young, ignorant, and makes her "first mistake" even though her mother may be far from pleased. Subsequent "mistakes," however, may be firmly dealt with--even to the point that a girl's mother will refuse to accept any more of her babies to raise, so that she is driven to seek abortion (Cf. #178, comment by informant 39).

9. Kin vs. non-kin

Kinship is a large subject in any culture or subculture, and I will not attempt to analyze the kinship system of the ghetto here in detail. There are, however, a few distinctive features which were noted in the course of the fieldwork, though only some are implied by the folklore *per se*, and these seem worthy of mention.

Kinship terminology is somewhat special, in that half-sisters and brothers who are children of the same mother are not likely to acknowledge the half-relationship, but think and speak of one another as brothers and sisters without qualifiers. Another kind of special usage conveys certain subtleties of mating arrangements. A husband (legal) is always referred to as "my husband"--but a man with whom one is living out of wedlock is referred to by other terms, as a rule. If the relationship is of long standing and there are several children, their father will usually be called "my old man." If there is less permanence in the arrangement, or if the couple do not live together, the woman will call her mate "my boyfriend."[5]

Despite careful avoidance of the inaccurate application of the term "husband," however, it was not uncommon for a woman to refer to her "old man's" or "boyfriend's" mother as "mother-in-law" and to other members of his family by equivalent in-law terms, particularly if the couple lived together. (Young girls still living at home were likelier to refer to "my boyfriend's mother.") Where a woman had been abandoned by her child's father, however, she never called him "my" anything--he was "the baby's father" and related to the child, but not to her.

Thus there is a scale of terms for the fathers of children which seems to denote the greater or lesser security of the woman's relationship to him. These may even be thought of as a hierarchy in which a legal husband, regardless of whether the marriage is a happy one, occupies the top place.

In a subcultural universe in which marriage is quite often brittle, and many children are born out of wedlock, the most enduring and important ties are those of blood. A woman's female consanguines are of particular importance, and it is of course commonplace that the incidence of two- and three-generation matrifocal households is high throughout the ghetto, just as it is among my particular group of informants. Even where my data indicate that a woman lives alone with her offspring, she frequently lives within a block or two of her mother or sister, who are readily available in emergencies. If a solidary kin group exists in the ghetto, it is the group of mother and daughters.

Less emphasized, but also important are relationships between in-law women. It is common to find that a married woman has entered into a kind of alliance with her mother-in-law and sisters-in-law, and that they are also an important solidarity in times of celebration or emergency. Two women, in fact, lived with a mother-in-law in preference to their own mothers, and several others moved to be nearer their in-law families. In-law relationships frequently survive importantly even after the break-up of a marriage.

There are fictive categories of kin, as well, in the ghetto. This subject has been dealt with by Liebow (1967) in some detail, and is confirmed by references made by my informants (usually those whose real kin were far away) to "my play mother" or "play sister."

The most important of all kin ties, however, is that between mother and child. This relationship is both unique ("you don't have but one mother in your lifetime") and permanent ("no matter what he done, he's always your child, and nothing can change that.") Because they are all children of the same mother, children are siblings--even though they might have different fathers. The gravest insult one person can offer another is one which mentions "your mother" in invidious terms, even though the same term can be employed in friendly contexts as a casual or jocular mode of address.[6]

10. Male vs. female

Here I will deal with conceptions of maleness and femaleness, rather than with the relationships between male and female, for which I lack data provided by males. Of course the conception which females have of the two sexes' innate characteristics are biassed, too, but since they are quite expressly implicit in both the lore and in more casual utterances they cannot be passed over as irrelevant here.

The expression of preference for a baby of one or the other sex was usual among my informants. Few women came out with the statement typical of white middle-class mothers: "I don't care what it is, as long as it's healthy." Not only was preference expressed before the baby's birth, in cases when the woman was interviewed at that time, but afterwards, when women were quite openly elated or disappointed over the newborn's sex. This happened even if they were older mothers who already had children of both sexes.

Patients were about evenly divided between those who wanted boys and those who wanted girls, so that there was no statistical bias toward either sex. What was most interesting, however, was the almost unanimous agreement on the reasons one might have for preferring one over the other, regardless of one's own personal preference.

Whether a woman preferred a boy or a girl, the women agreed that boys were "less trouble" in terms of physical care. The trouble factor seemed to center around the fact that boys were easier and cheaper to dress adequately, and took less in terms of grooming. As one informant put it, "You can put a boy in a T-shirt and a pair of dungarees and send them out in the street to play. But a girl--you got to comb their hair, wash their dresses and iron them--somehow you got to keep a little girl cleaner." On this basis a mother of a large family might prefer the new baby to be born a boy, since there was less of a physical burden imposed by boys in the early years (Cf. #274, 275).

On the other hand, boys were seen as presenting more behavior problems than girls. They were more apt to be rough and destructive, as well as more difficult to control than girls. Girls, moreover, "stay close to you when they're grown" whereas boys are likely to wander off--another sign, obviously, that the intergenerational solidarity of women is much stronger than that of men or that between men and women (Cf. #273). Thus, while a little girl is "more trouble" in early childhood--mainly because her hair must be laboriously combed and braided up each day--the investment of time and effort, and the expense of clothing a little girl properly seemed worthwhile to most women at least once in a lifetime because girls are more tractable and rewarding as they grow up. Ideally a family has children of both sexes, and "a boy and a girl is a rich man's family" (Cf. #269). Most mothers, therefore, would like at least "one little girl to raise" because even if she's "more trouble" she is also "fun to dress up all pretty," and is likelier to bring emotional satisfactions to the mother.

These attitudes toward male and female children are not so straightforward as they might seem on the surface, however, and I would be inclined to discount somewhat the "trouble" factor as the whole reason for sexual preferences.

Several investigators have noted as a lower-class phenomenon the lack of real psychological intimacy between the sexes, and the strict division which generally obtains between men's and women's work and leisure activities.[7] The interplay of the sexes in adult life among the poor generally, and among my informants in particular, may well be such that there is real ambivalence among women toward having male children at all--an ambivalence which is only partially resolved through the rationalization that boys, at least when they are small, are "easier." The solidary nature of female consanguineal groups, too, would tend to support this interpretation.

In addition to the amount of "trouble" the two sexes are to the mother, they are viewed as having innate differences of temperament and behavior. Boys are inclined to be rough and less amenable to discipline, therefore "badder" than girls as well as likelier to end in trouble with society, including serious trouble with police. They are even "rougher" while in utero (Cf. #27, 30) in the view of several informants. On the other hand, they are thought to be "lazy" and even "slow"--also characteristics which may be manifested before birth (Cf. #31, 153) and which are seen as reasons they are "harder to train."

Girls, too, present a specific constellation of traits thought of as female. They are, indeed, prettier and more fun to dress than boys, but they also present a mother with a certain degree of anxiety when they reach puberty, when they must be carefully supervised and educated lest they become pregnant (Cf. #63, 276). This, of course, is an ideal formulation often breached in practice, to judge by the number of very young girls with illegitimate children. In any case, since girls are generally more help around the house, stick closer to home and are more obedient and affectionate, it seemed that on balance girls were the preferred sex for reasons other than practical ones related to early care.

Adult men are supposed to be strong and tough, ideally, in keeping with the temperament thought innate to males and manifest throughout the male life cycle, even before birth. Even so, they are conceived of as weak in certain respects--particularly as fathers in the role of breadwinners, and with reference to their general self-esteem. (The two are, of course, quite probably connected, since the breadwinner role is the central paternal role in U. S. culture at large.) A woman, if she has a husband whom she loves, must therefore be careful, in order to maintain a happy family life, not to "mess up a man's pride" by being suspect as to her faithfulness or by failing to give in to him in small matters (Cf. #264 through 266). Basically a man may be neither affectionate toward his family nor terribly competent with children (Cf. #267, 268)--but if you love him you put up with him.

Adult women are, first and foremost, cut out to be mothers, both biologically and temperamentally. Motherhood is both a joy and a trial, as it is elsewhere in American culture, but it is, regardless of the mix of pleasure and pain, the central feminine role without which a woman is not complete. Mother love is the strongest of all loves, and the most enduring.

To some extent pregnancy is a time of privilege during which women are allowed to be somewhat unstable, whimsical and self-indulgent, as has already been noted in the discussion of autonomy vs. dependence (Cf. pp. 92-95). Newman believes that pregnancy is "a period of regression of the woman to an infantile state approximating that of the fetus within her" (1965:56) and sees it as a state of exaggerated dependence, rather than a period of willfulness or autonomous behavior, as I have characterized it. Nevertheless, whichever way one chooses to look at it, pregnancy is the period which brings most strongly into play a female's pride in her own fertility, her solidarity with other child-bearing females, and her underlying sense of moral superiority to men. (Thus, "If men had to have the babies, there wouldn't be any children in the world.")

11. Nurturance vs. Deprivation

Although breast feeding is traditionally believed to be the "best thing for the baby" (Cf. #151) it was practiced by only two of my informants, and was overtly viewed with revulsion or shame by at least six (Cf. #151 comments, and #280). Newman (1965) has suggested that in American culture generally the breast is a focus of value-conflict, because it simultaneously symbolizes both eroticism and maternal nurture. Since this double meaning of the breast implies conflict between maternal and conjugal roles, and since the conflict is rather easily resolved by giving babies bottles, women tend to opt for the conjugal role.

If Newman's interpretation is correct, it would seem that the behavior of my informants in this respect is quite in keeping with that of most other Americans. Indeed, since it is less rational economically for lower class mothers to bottle feed, due to the expense, there may also be an element here, as elsewhere, of lower class emulation of middle class consumption patterns.

Despite the fact that breast feeding has nearly disappeared from the ghetto, however, feeding is still the maternal act, and as such it is of vital symbolic importance. A mother must always feed her own child, even if he is left in the care of someone else while she works during the day. It is standard practice, for example, for children who must be fed away from home to have their food brought with them from home to the place where they are being care for. A woman who permits her child to eat casually in the homes of playmates is likely to become the subject of much malicious gossip, for it is assumed that if she allows this she must be short of food at home, and to let children go hungry is disgraceful.[8]

Food is the most important expression of maternal love, so that the criticism which is leveled at mothers whose children go hungry goes quite beyond mere speculation about their financial solvency. Even if she has to steal to do it, a mother is obligated to feed her children, for this is the expression of her feeling for them. Indeed, since other open expressions of affection and other kinds of giving are feared as likely to "spoil" children, (Cf. #148, 149, 277, 278) food and love are nearly coextensive. Thus the mothers on the ward were much preoccupied with the quality and amount of formula brought for them to feed their babies in the hospital, and several pronounced it wanting and vowed to give their babies something "with more body to it" when they took them home (Cf. #224, 225). That this attitude sometimes results in overfeeding seems probable (Cf. #143).

There is probably a connection between the emphasis on feeding and the great pride taken in babies who were born big and fat. Conversely, mothers of premature or otherwise puny offspring were chagrined and somewhat apologetic, as though their own mothering capabilities were under criticism even at the moment of birth. One rationalized that "small babies grow faster . . . because they got to catch up," presumably to console herself for her own infant's puniness. (This, incidentally, is a general part of American lore and was told to me at the birth of my own first child. Cf. #152).

Other aspects of nurture were less important than feeding, but were also mentioned. Women laid particular emphasis, for example, on dressing children nicely and keeping them clean, especially when they take them out on the street to be seen by others. The implication is that a mother will be judged by the outward appearance of her children, therefore, women take a good deal of pleasure in buying them pretty clothes--especially if they are girl children (Cf. #274, 275, 279). This area, so much taken for granted at upper levels of U. S. society that it can be treated negligently, is probably important throughout the lower class, and not peculiar only to the black lower class.

Conspicuously absent, for the most part, as an intrinsic part of maternal nurture, is education in the formal sense. One has a responsibility to teach children to "behave" (which here as elsewhere tends to mean teaching them not to annoy or embarrass adults) and girls are taught to help out in the home when they are "old enough" but most other kinds of teaching are thought to be the province of the schools. Although mothers with school age children are freely (and quite often penetratingly) critical of schools and teachers for failing to make children "behave" in school so that they can learn, they do not conceive it as their nurturant role to supplement school fare in the home. Hard worked as many of these mothers are, this is probably not surprising, but it is interesting that even such items as crayons are likely to be barred from the home because children might mark up walls with them. This creates extra trouble for the mother, who has to spend all her time keeping everyone fed, washed and ironed. This, of course, is hardly an accurately descriptive statement for every informant--but it does indicate accurately, I believe, the way in which the value hierarchy is arranged: it is more important to avoid mess and dirt in the house than to allow children certain learning experiences. Here, too, the women of the ghetto are far from unique.

During her pregnancy a woman is supposed to display nurturing concern for the unborn child. She should, therefore, guard herself against overwork, falls, frights and other hazards to the infant's welfare *in utero* so that it will not be born fragile or disfigured (Cf. #94, 95, 104, 107, 108, 109, 112, 114, 116). Some of these beliefs, of course, can cut both ways, in that a girl who is impatient with waiting can surreptitiously engage in activities designed to bring on labor, or even miscarriage (Cf. #98, as well as the case of Margaret, pp. 82-83). No one, however, hinted in any way that they would have deliberately tried to cause any disfigurement through the breaking of taboos on a pregnant woman's activities. If one is going to have a baby, obviously one wishes it to be normal physically.

In summary, then, nurturance and deprivation are seen as hinging largely on the matter of physical care, with special importance given to feeding and somewhat less (but still a good deal) to clothing and cleanliness. A mother who is obviously derelict in her duty in these major areas is subject to malicious gossip, and women become very defensive if they are not able to keep up at least an outward appearance of taking good care of their offspring in these respects. Children are likely to be punished, in fact, for begging food of others, for dirtying their clothes or for tearing them because this publicly reflects upon the mother's care. Ideally, too, a pregnant woman displays intense concern for the unborn child and practices numerous avoidances (though few positive measures) to insure its welfare. There is a tacit admission however that not all taboos are equally important, and that the comfort of the mother may at times take precedence, so that observance of them varies with the individual. In any case it is less serious to neglect an unborn child than to fail in one's duty to those already here--one may even hope secretly that the baby will miscarry through some "innocent" oversight on the mother's part, though one would never seek to harm a living child. Once a baby is born alive a mother's love for it comes into play, so that she is bound to do her best for it.

12. <u>Legitimate vs. illegitimate</u>

The terms employed for this category are truly the anthropologist's categories, for no woman interviewed ever referred to her own or anyone else's child as "illegitimate." Here, perhaps, is the area of greatest contrast between the categories adhered to by most other Americans and those which exist in the ghetto subculture. There are "women who has babies without being married," and they may even be gossiped about if they are otherwise unpopular for some reason, but there are no "illegitimate" babies, and the term "bastard" is hurled at mothers, not at children, when women quarrel. Such criticism as exists is leveled at the mother alone, and the child is in no way stigmatized by his mother's behavior, even though he may be pitied if others regard him as neglected by a woman who is "nothing but an old sow" (i.e., really promiscuous, with numerous children by different men).

Such criticism is, in any case, usually reserved for extreme cases, and a girl's "first mistake" is generally tolerated without much comment outside her own family. This does not mean that the first pregnancy out of wedlock is viewed lightly by either the girl or her own parents, however, for it may be both a personal and a family calamity in emotional and practical terms. If the girl is very young she may be ill-prepared for motherhood and resentful of the numerous changes in her life that the new role will entail. Her own mother (and father, if one is present) may be barely managing to subsist and worried about the added burden on the family budget. Nevertheless, a girl will seldom be forced into marriage if she is very young, particularly if the father of her child is also very young and doesn't earn a living, or if he comes from a family the girl's family feels to be "no good." Indeed, even if the girl wants to marry the boy her own mother may refuse to allow it until she is pregnant for a second time. There were three such cases known to me among my informants.

It seems fair to state, however, that there is virtually no social or moral pressure within the ghetto for a girl either to marry precipitately or to place her baby for adoption, and both situations seem to be rare. The possible reason for this distinctive development of the black subculture in this country has been speculated upon by numerous authors as being due to the history of slavery, to the economically marginal position of Negro men, or even, in a racist context, to the inherent moral inferiority of Negroes. A more sophisticated recent explanation has been outlined by Whitten and Szwed, who suggest that the family as we know it may be dysfunctional in ghetto conditions, and that the integration of black communities may be based upon individual networks of opportunistic and flexible affiliations rather than on kin ties. This makes legal marriage functionally superfluous (1970:NYP).

Whatever the reasons for its existence, the obliteration of the distinction between legitimate and illegitimate children which is so rigidly in effect in the mainstream U. S. culture is a primary distinguishing feature of the ghetto subculture. Since there is little or no moral pressure on mothers to give such children up, we find here a further explanation for the extreme censure which has been mentioned elsewhere as attending the placement of a child for adoption. Since society (or this segment of it) does not stigmatize the mother very seriously or the child at all, only a woman who totally rejects the feminine maternal role could do such a thing. Such a woman is viewed as an unnatural creature indeed, and the pressures upon a girl who has thus adopted the values of the larger world is considerable, even punitive.

The Ghetto Subculture

An underlying assumption of the present study has been, as was stated at the outset, that the Negro women who have been its subjects are, in some sense, representative of a distinctive subculture within American society. It is perhaps appropriate here to examine this assumption further, and to outline briefly the major positions of students of the American Negro.

The empirical distinctiveness of the life style -- or perhaps more properly the several life styles -- of northern urban ghettoes does not appear to be much debated. Further, it is generally agreed that many of the poor and black living in our cities display patterns of behavior which not only differ markedly, but in quite predictable ways from those of the American mainstream. Thus there seems to be little dispute about the fact that my subjects belong to a behaviorally distinctive sub-group within U. S. society. What is at issue, and what has given rise to much acrimonious debate, is the manner in which one may interpret the empirical facts. In brief, the argument seems to center around the issue of whether or not this sub-*group* also possesses or belongs to a sub*culture*. Is the life of the ghetto expressive of social pathology, an unorganized or disorganized way of life, or has it a system of symbols which is distinctively its own and which sanctions behavior which the mainstream culture sees only as "deviant?"

Valentine (1968) has eloquently criticized the current "intellectual fad" which ascribes cultures or subcultures to almost any social category, and maintains that this fad not only distorts the whole concept of culture, but leads to pernicious misconceptions concerning the nature of and remedies for many social problems, particularly that of poverty. In particular, he attacks Lewis's (1966) "culture of poverty" concept--although it should perhaps be noted that Lewis was hardly the first to attribute distinctive subcultures to different social classes.

With respect to the black slum dweller and his empirically distinctive patterns of behavior, we find that there are several alternative explanations of the observed phenomena. At least two distinct polarities and a possible mediating position may be distinguished for present purposes--though this is by no means an exhaustive listing of the many interpretations which have been placed on ghetto life.

At one pole stand those investigators who view either (a) the poverty or (b) the African heritage of the U. S. Negro as having produced a unique set of patterns for living which are relatively stable, enduring and positively valued within the ghetto community. Lewis is frequently associated with the former view, although his formulation (Cf. Lewis, 1966) hesitates to include groups within the modern "welfare state" in the "culture of poverty" typology at all. Herskovits (1941) was the earliest and most thorough scientific exponent of the second. In any case, both wings of investigators occupy what I shall refer to as the "cultural" position. Further, ghetto culture (or more strictly "subculture") is viewed in a very traditional anthropological fashion as being very persistent and rather conservative. One possible implication of this view is that neither full integration into U. S. society nor the elimination of poverty is likely to do away with either the distinctive ghetto pattern of behavior, or the "social problems" (in the larger society's terms, and possibly also in the ghetto-dweller's as well) which arise from it. Presumably, therefore, the patterns to which such a subculture gives rise must be accepted as one of a plurality of patterns which are to be found within the society as a whole.

At the other pole stand those investigators who view the distinctive features of ghetto life as nothing more than a set of situational adaptations, neither positively valued nor socially transmitted, and therefore not "cultural" at all. These patterns are, rather, seen as a series of <u>ad hoc</u> responses to the social exclusion and economic deprivation of blacks within our society. This set of responses is somehow monotonously rediscovered by each generation as it grows to maturity in similar depressed circumstances in the ghetto. It is not, however, a style of life to which ghetto people feel real attachment, for it is one which merely reiterates and reinforces feelings of failure as they compare the reality of their lives with the standards held up by the larger society. The most outspoken recent exponent of this position, which I shall call the "situational" position, is Liebow (1967)--but he is only the most recent heir to a position earlier stated by Frazier and often reiterated since.

The implication of this view, in which the ghetto dweller is seen as existing with a sense of chronic failure in a forced adaptation to poverty and exclusion, is that ghetto society is, indeed, pathologically disorganized and lacking in coherent values and norms of its own. From a policy standpoint, however, things look brighter--for if this is the case, all the "social problems" which this group generates for white society can easily be cured by means of large infusions of money and the integration of blacks into the socioeconomic system as full and equal citizens.

A third view of the situation is based on a conception of culture which differs somewhat in its basic assumptions from those which are implicit in the other two views. Instead of culture being viewed as a consciously valued and transmitted set of patterns for living which an elder generation hands down to a younger one, this view "emphasizes the sharing of cultural imagery, of expectations and definitions of reality, as the medium whereby individuals in a community interact" (Hannerz, 1969: 21)--regardless, it might be added, of generation. As to the matter of whether or not there is such a thing as a ghetto-specific culture, this will "obviously . . . depend to some extent on what we shall mean by culture."

Hannerz believes that in the ghetto we can observe both "mainstream" and "ghetto specific" cultures, and points to the heterogeneity of behavioral styles, both as these styles vary between individuals, and as they may occur within the context of a single life career. Attachment to one or the other culture, furthermore, seems to vary widely with both situations and personalities. As to the policy implications of his view, Hannerz rather weakly proposes that perhaps "social policy, in some areas, may well proceed unaffected by the questions raised by a ghetto-specific culture." One gathers from this statement that social policy may, regardless of the existence of a true subculture of ghetto people, proceed on the assumption that ghetto dwellers' goals, aspirations and needs are no different than anyone else's, and that therefore the solutions to their problems need be no different. Indeed, one need not even, one supposes, consult them as to what their problems, as they perceive them, really are.

Hannerz has, however, given needed attention to the data which indicate, as I have tried to do earlier as well, the wide variety of adjustments present in the ghetto, which do not yield to simplistic either-or formulations of either the "cultural" or the "situational" variety. He also recalls us to a very venerable fundamental of anthropological theory which is often submerged in the partisan debate. This is, that culture is in a very important sense, situationally adaptive, so that there is really no inherent contradiction between the cultural and situational positions at all. Behavior does, indeed, change all the time in adaptation to changing conditions of many sorts, but this does not at all obviate the probability that such behavioral change will acquire cultural support in the form of appropriate symbols, perceptions of the world, and values. The cultural guides to behavior, in their turn, tend to be persistent--to lag, perhaps, behind behavioral change, or to slow down the rate of such change in some instances.

It is this view which I find most reasonable in the light of my own data. My informants do not behave either like automatons in the grip of blind cultural tradition, nor like the players of some zero-sum game in which they seek only to maximize their own advantage. In short, like other human beings, their behavior indicates the presence of both rational and irrational forces at work in their lives, and is informed neither by the purely adaptive values of games theory nor by some selfless loyalty to dysfunctional ways of life.

With Hannerz, I would maintain that both "mainstream culture" and "ghetto-specific culture" influence life in the ghetto. At times the effect created is of a kind of oscillation between the two, and at other times the effect seems closer to what Rodman called "the lower-class value stretch" (1965). The latter situation has been aptly described by Suttles as existing among slum dwellers of all colors, and as one in which "conventional social norms are not rejected, but emphasized differently or suspended for established reasons . . . (while) those who remain in good standing are often exceptionally tolerant of and even encouraging to those who are 'deviant'" (1969:16).

That the very heterogeneous picture of ghetto life and culture may be a consequence of competing values as much as of stretched ones cannot be discounted as a possibility. What is certain, however, is that the situation is one which is enormously complex--one in which tradition and adaptive behavior continuously modify one another, one in which "black values" and "mainstream aspirations" exist in dynamic tension, one in which the term "social problem" is in need of cautious definition. The present study can hardly begin to give any definitive answers to the way in which all these variables interact, but there is hope, perhaps, that these questions can be clarified through further, more sophisticated and more sensitive inquiries into the lives and the subcultures of the urban ghetto.

FOOTNOTES--CHAPTER VII

[1]The notion of "legitimacy" for example, may have political as well as legal or moral implications, and may refer to the basis for an entire power structure, as when we ask the question "who is a legitimate leader in this society?" Here, however, I restrict its meaning to the matter of bastardy, since wider inferences cannot be made from the present corpus.

[2]I refer here to early adolescents, in the main. The seventeen or eighteen year old high school girl whose friends may all be having babies and who may feel that she, too, must have one in order to validate her status as a mature female is a different sort of case. I have no specific data from my own informants, but other sources (Abrahams, 1964:27, and two Philadelphia high school teachers) suggest that girls in their late teens may want a baby, whether or not they are eager to marry, and surely know how one goes about having one by the time they have reached this age.

[3]One cannot, for example, move about freely, particularly across state lines, if one receives public assistance, because many states require a year's residence before one becomes eligible. A woman who is unable to work is therefore effectively restricted, if she has no employable husband, from leaving the state in which she is eligible. Until recently, of course, her sex life, too, was subject to regulation under public assistance codes which made any man living in the house responsible for a family's support, whether or not her children are his.

It is possible to speculate that the lack of economic autonomy which is so prevalent in the ghetto may be a source of compensatory values, such as the ability to "cheat the welfare people" and the appearance of the "hustler" as a kind of culture-hero.

[4]On the other hand, a few mothers admitted, with an air of pride, that they "spoil" their children through indulging their own soft-hearted motherly love. Thus, "spoiling" is occasionally seen in a positive light, and not as an absolute evil, though it will always make children more troublesome to raise.

[5]See Liebow (1967) for his discussion of very similar findings among low-income Negroes in Washington, D. C.

[6]Cf. Abrahams, 1964, whose collection of tales is freely sprinkled with both the insulting and the casual use of the term "motherfucker" among Negro males. The term was not used by my informants, however, either to me or in my hearing among themselves.

[7]See Liebow (1967) in which the contrast between male-female relationships, which are stormy and exploitive, and friendships between males, which are solidary, is discussed at length. Cf. also Gans (1968) and Abrahams (1964:20) who discuss the separation of men's and women's worlds, as does Komarovsky (1962) in her book on lower-class marriage.

[8] The system described here was observed in action in the home of an elderly woman at Raymond Rosen Projects, who regularly babysat for several small children from different families, while their mothers worked. Each morning the mothers brought their children to Mrs. B's home, along with sufficient food for their lunch and snacks during the day. No child was fed the food belonging to another--even so much as a cookie--and mothers who were a bit short on any given day were quite defensive and apologetic, and were gossiped about in their absence. Slurring remarks were also made about other children in the project who tended to "drop in" at mealtimes, although they were never refused food, which Mrs. B used to supply from her own small store of edibles.

BIBLIOGRAPHY

Abrahams, Roger D. A Rhetoric of Everyday Life: Traditional Conversational Genres. University of Texas, n.d.

_______. Negro Folklore from South Philadelphia: A Collection and Analysis. Unpublished Ph.D. dissertation, University of Pennsylvania, 1962.

_______. Deep Down in the Jungle: Negro Narrative. Folklore from the Streets of Philadelphia. Hatboro: Folklore Associates, 1964.

Banton, Michael. ASA 3: Anthropological Approaches to the Study of Religion. London: Tavistock, 1966.

Bascom, William R. "Four Functions of Folklore." Journal of American Folklore, 67: 333-349 (1954).

_______. "Folklore and Anthropology." Journal of American Folklore, 66:283-290 (1953).

Bartlett, F., et al. The Study of Society: Methods and Problems. New York: Macmillan, 1939.

Bauman, Richard. "Y. L. Cahan's Instructions on the Collecting of Folklore." New York Folklore Quarterly, 18:284-289 (1962).

Ben Amos, Dan. "Folklore: The Definition Game Once Again." Paper read at meetings of the American Folklore Society, Toronto, 1967.

Benedict, Ruth. "Folklore." Encyclopedia of the Social Sciences. New York: Macmillan, 1937, pp. 288-93.

_______. Patterns of Culture. New York: Houghton Mifflin, 1934.

Bennett, J. W. "The Study of Cultures: A Survey of Technique and Methodology in Fieldwork." American Sociological Review, 13:672-689 (1948).

Bernard, Jessie. Marriage and Family Among Negroes. Englewood Cliffs, N. J.: Prentice-Hall, 1966.

Bieber, Toby Bennett. A Comparison Study of Negro Wed and Unwed Mothers. Unpublished Ph.D. dissertation, Columbia University, 1964.

Boas, Franz. Anthropology. New York: Columbia University Press, 1908.

Botkin, B. A. Lay My Burden Down: A Folk History of Slavery. Chicago: University of Chicago Press, 1945.

Brendle, Thomas R., and Unger, Claude W. Folk Medicine of the Pennsylvania Germans: The Non-Occult Cures. Norristown, Pa.: Pennsylvania German Society, 1935.

Brown, Frank C. North Carolina Folklore. Durham: Duke University Press, 1952-64.

Browne, Ray. Popular Beliefs and Bractices from Alabama. Berkeley: University of California Press, 1958.

Brunson, Rose. Socialization Experience and Socioeconomic Characteristics of Urban Negroes as Related to Use of Selected Southern Foods and Medical Remedies. Unpublished Ph.D. dissertation, University of Michigan, 1962.

Burke, Kenneth. The Philosophy of Literary Form. New York: Random House, 1941.

Butcher, Margaret Just. The Negro in American Culture. New York: New American Library, 1959.

Cameron, Vivian Knowles. Folk Beliefs Pertaining to the Health of American Negroes. Unpublished M.A. thesis, Northwestern University, 1930.

Campbell, Marie. Folks Do Get Born. New York: Rinehart, 1946.

Chilman, Catherine S. Growing Up Poor. U. S. Department of Health, Education and Welfare, Welfare Administration Division of Research, U. S. Government Printing Office, 1966.

Coult, Allan D. "Unconscious Inference and Cultural Origins." American Anthropologist, 65:32-35 (1963).

Davidson, Levette J. A Guide to American Folklore. Denver: Sage Books, 1951.

Dean, John P., and Whyte, William Foote. "How Do You Know the Informant is Telling the Truth?" Human Organization, 17:34-39 (1958).

Diaz, May N. Tonala: Conservatism, Responsibility and Authority in a Mexican Town. Berkeley: University of California Press, 1966.

Dorson, Richard M. American Negro Folktales. Greenwich, Conn.: Fawcett Publications, 1956.

Douglas, Mary. Purity and Danger. New York: Praeger, 1966.

Drake, Donald C. "OB-GYN at Temple Hospital: Doctor Lights Candle in Ghetto's Darkness." Philadelphia Inquirer, April 27, 1969.

Dundes, Alan. "Brown County Superstitions: The Structure of Superstition." Midwest Folklore, XI:25-56 (1961).

______. The Study of Folklore. Englewood Cliffs, N. J.: Prentice-Hall, 1965.

______. "On the Psychology of Collecting Folklore." Tennessee Folk Society Bulletin #28:65-74 (1962).

Eddington, Neil. The Urban Plantation: An Ethnology of an Oral Tradition. Unpublished Ph.D. dissertation, Berkeley, 1968.

Eisenstadt, S. "Anthropological Studies of Complex Societies." Current Anthropology, 2:201-222 (1961).

Evans-Pritchard, E. E. "Fieldwork and the Empirical Tradition." In Social Anthropology. London: Coben and West, 1951.

Ferman, Louis A., Kornbluh, Joyce L., and Haber, Alan. Poverty in America. Ann Arbor: University of Michigan Press, 1965.

Ford, Clellan S. Field Guide to the Study of Human Reproduction. New Haven: HRAF Press, 1964.

Frye, Christopher, Kluckhohn, Clyde, and Wigglesworth, V.B. Three Lectures. Toronto: University of Toronto, 1958.

Fox, Robin. Kinship and Marriage. Baltimore: Penguin Books, 1967.

Gans, Herber J. "Subculture and Class." In Ferman, et al., Poverty in America. Ann Arbor: University of Michigan Press, 1965.

Geertz, Clifford. "Form and Variation in Balinese Village Structure." American Anthropologist, 61:991-1012 (1959).

Goddard, P. E. "The Relation of Folklore to Anthropology." Journal of American Folklore, 28:18-23 (1915).

Goffman, Erving. The Presentation of Self in Everyday Life. Garden City, New York: Doubleday, 1959.

______. Asylums. Garden City, N. Y.: Doubleday, 1961.

Goldstein, Kenneth S. A Guide for Fieldworkers in Folklore. Hatboro: Folklore Associates, 1964.

______. "The Collecting of Superstitious Beliefs." Keystone Folklore Quarterly, 9:13-22 (1964).

Gorer, Goeffry. Himalayan Village. London: St. Joseph, 1938.

Halpert, Herbert. "The Functional Approach." In Conference on the Character and State of Studies in Folklore, Journal of American Folklore, 59: 510-512 (1946).

______. "Some Undeveloped Areas in American Folklore." Journal of American Folklore, 70:299-304 (1957).

Hand, Wayland D. "American Analogues of the Couvade." In Richmond, Studies in Folklore. Bloomington: Indiana University Press, 1957.

Hannerz, Ulf. "Roots of Black Manhood." Trans-Action, October, 1969:13-21.

Henry, Jules. Culture Against Man. New York: Random House, 1963.

Herskovits, Melville J. The Myth of the Negro Past. Boston: Beacon Press, 1941.

______. "The Hypothetical Situation: A Technique of Field Research." Southwestern Journal of Anthropology, 6:32-40 (1950).

Homans, George C. "Anxiety and Ritual: The Theories of Malinowsi and Radcliffe-Brown." American Anthropologist, XLIII:164-72 (1941).

Honko, Lauri. "Memorates and the Study of Folk Beliefs." Journal of the Folklore Institute, 1:5-19 (1968).

Horowitz, Michael M. "A Decision Model of Conjugal Patterns in Martinique." Man, 2:445-453 (1967).

Irelan, Lola M. "Health Practices of the Poor." In Low Income Life Styles. U. S. Department of Health, Education, and Welfare, U. S. Government Printing Office, Washington, D. C., 1967.

Jackson, Bruce (ed). The Negro and His Folklore in Nineteenth Century Periodicals. Austin: American Folklore Society, University of Texas Press, 1967.

Jahoda, Marie, Deutsch, Morton, and Cook, Stuart W. (eds.). Research Methods in Social Relations. New York: Dryden Press, 1951.

Kelly, Isabel Truesdell. Folk Practices in North Mexico. Austin: Institute of Latin American Studies, University of Texas Press, 1965.

King, Lewis. Negro Life in a Rural Community. Unpublished Ph.D. dissertation, Columbia University, 1965.

Kluckhohn, Clyde. "The Scientific Study of Values." In Frye, Kluckhohn, and Wigglesworth, Three Lectures. Toronto: University of Toronto, 1958.

Kochman, Thomas. "Rapping in the Black Ghetto." Trans-Action, February, 1969:26-34.

Komarovsky, Mirra. Blue Collar Marriage. New York: Random House, 1962.

Kunstadter, Peter. "A Survey of the Consanguine or Matrifocal Family." American Anthropologist, 65:56-66 (1963).

Leo, John. "Sociology Scored by Negro Leader." New York Times, August 28, 1968.

Lesser, Alexander. "Superstition." Journal of Philosophy, 1931.

Levi-Strauss, Claude. The Savage Mind. Chicago: University of Chicago Press, 1966.

Levy, M. J., Jr., and Fallers, L. A. "The Family: Some Comparative Considerations." American Anthropologist, 61:647-451 (1959).

Lewis, Oscar. "The Culture of Poverty." Scientific American, October, 1966.

Liebow, Elliot. Talley's Corner: A Study of Negro Streetcorner Men. Boston: Little, Brown and Company, 1967.

Lomax, Alan. "The Functional Aspects of Folklore." In Conference on the Character and State of Studies in Folklore, Journal of American Folklore, 59:507-510 (1946).

Lowie, Robert. Ethnologist. Berkeley: University of California Press, 1959.

Malinowski, Bronislaw. "Myth in Primitive Psychology." In Magic Science and Religion. New York: Doubleday, 1948.

_______. "The Group and the Individual in Functional Analysis." American Journal of Sociology, XLIV: 938-964.

McBroom, Patricia. "The Black Matriarchy: Healthy or Pathological?" Science News, October 19, 1968: 393-395.

Mead, Margaret. "The Effects of Anthropological Fieldwork Models on Interdisciplinary Communication." Journal of Social Issues, II:3-11 (1955).

_______. "Appendix." In New Lives for Old. New York: Morrow, 1956.

Miller, Walter B. "Focal Concerns of Lower-Class Culture." In Ferman, et al., Poverty in America. Ann Arbor: University of Michigan Press, 1965.

Nadel, S. F. "The Interview Technique in Social Anthropology." In Bartlett, et al (eds.), The Study of Society. New York: Macmillan, 1939.

Newman, Lucile F. Culture and Perinatal Development in American Society. Unpublished Ph.D. dissertation, University of California at Berkeley, 1965.

Opler, Morris E. "The Human Being in Culture Theory." American Anthropologist, 66:507-528 (1964).

Passin, Herbert, and Bennett, John W. "Changing Agricultural Magic in Southern Illinois: A Systematic Analysis of Folk-Urban Transmission." In Dundes (ed.), The Study of Folklore. Englewood Cliffs, N. J.: Prentice-Hall, 1965.

Paul, Benjamin D. "Interview Techniques and Field Relationships." In Tax (ed)., Anthropology Today.

Powdermaker, Hortense. Stranger and Friend. New York: W. W. Norton, 1966.

Puckett, Newbell Niles. Folk Beliefs of the Southern Negro. Chapel Hill: University of North Carolina Press, 1926.

Randolph, Vance. Ozark Superstitions. New York: Columbia University Press, 1947.

Redfield, Robert. The Primitive World and Its Transformations. Ithaca: Cornell University Press, 1953.

Richmond, W. E. (ed). Studies in Folklore. Bloomington: Indiana University Press, 1957.

Rodman, Hyman. "The Lower-Class Value Stretch." In Ferman, et al., Poverty in America. Ann Arbor: University of Michigan Press, 1965.

Schneider, David. American Kinship: A Cultural Account. Englewood Cliffs, N. J.: Prentice-Hall, 1968.

Sebeok, Thomas A. Style in Language. Cambridge, Mass.: M.I.T. Press, 1960.

Seitel, Peter. "The Social Usage of Metaphor." Genre, II, No. 2 (1969).

Signor, Roger. "Anemia Plagues Rich and Poor." The Philadelphia Inquirer, December 22, 1968.

Simpson, George. "Folk Medicine in Trinidad." Journal of American Folklore, 75: 326-40 (1962).

Smith, R. T. "Culture and Social Structure in the Caribbean: Some Recent Work on Family and Kinship Studies." Comparative Studies in Society and History, 6:24-46 (1962).

Spiro, M. E. "Religion: Problems of Definition and Explanation." In Banton, ASA 3, 1966.

Suttles, Gerald D. "Anatomy of a Chicago Slum." Trans-Action, February, 1969.

Thoms, William. "Folklore." In Dundes (ed)., The Study of Folklore. Englewood

Cliffs, N. J.: Prentice-Hall, 1965.

Utley, Francis Lee. "Folk Literature: An Operational Definition." In Dundes (ed)., The Study of Folklore. Englewood Cliffs, N. J.: Prentice-Hall, 1965.

U. S. Census Bureau. Statistical Abstracts of the United States for 1968. U. S. Government Printing Office, Washington, D. C., 1968.

Valentine, Charles. Culture and Poverty. Chicago: University of Chicago Press, 1968.

Voegelin, C. F. "Casual and Non-Casual Utterances within A Unified Structure." In Sebeok (ed)., Style in Language. Cambridge, Mass.: M.I.T. Press, 1960.

Wallace, Anthony F. K. Culture and Personality. New York: Random House, 1961.

Whitten, Norman, and Szwed, John F. "Introduction" to Afro-American Anthropology: Contemporary Perspectives. New York: Free Press, 1970.

_______. "Anthropologists Look at Afro-Americans." Trans-Action, July-August, 1968.

Wilson, Peter J. "Reputation and Respectability: A Suggestion for Caribbean Ethnology." Man, 4: 70-84 (1969).

APPENDIX A

CITY OF PHILADELPHIA
COMMUNITY HEALTH SERVICES
MATERNAL AND INFANT CARE PROJECT

INCOME LIMITS

Single, divorced or separated woman:		
Gross annual income up to		$3150 (+ Fetus)
+1	minor	3900
+2	minors	4650
+3	minors	5400
+4	minors	6100
+5	minors	6900

Married woman living with husband:		
Combined gross annual income up to		$4590 (+ Fetus)
+1	minor	5340
+2	minors	6090
+3	minors	6840
+4	minors	7590
+5	minors	8340

ADD $750.00 for each minor over 5

APPENDIX B

TABLE OF INFORMANTS WITH DATA PERTINENT TO STUDY

Key to Table:

Unreg:	Unregistered at clinic, therefore not eligible for aid.
NYD:	Not Yet Delivered
C. U.:	Concensual Union
BF:	Mate referred to by term other than "husband" (usually "boyfriend")
DPA:	Public Assistance
MIC:	City-administered aid to needy health-district families.

Code No.	Birth-place	Yrs. In. Urban N.	Age	Mar. Status	Years of School
1	Phila.	15	15	S	8
2	Phila.	23	23	Sep.	12
3	Phila.	17	17	S	11
4	N. J.	2	18	M	12
5	Phila.	20	20	S	12
6	N. C.	29	32	M	12
7	Chicago	21	21	M	11
8	N. C.	8	28	M	12
9	S. C.	17	34	M	?
10	Phila.	21	21	M	11
11	Phila.	24	24	M	11
12	Va.	2	17	Sep.	10
13	Fla.	30	32	C. U.	8
14	Ala.	9	28	S	12
15	Chester, Pa.	4	21	M	12
16	Phila.	17	17	S	11
17	Fla.	13	26	M	13
18	Phila.	25	25	C. U.	11
19	Fla.	1	18	M	9
20	Miss.	13	31	Sep.	7
21	Ga.	?	16	S	11
22	Phila.	16	16	S	9
23	Phila.	25	25	M	?
24	Chicago	7	23	S	10
25	Phila.	24	24	S	?
26	Phila.	20	20	C. U.	12
27	?	?	23	Sep.	?
28	Phila.	6	19	S	13
29	Phila.	23	23	C. U.	12
30	Phila.	25	25	C. U.	11
31	Phila.	16	22	S	10
32	Phila.	42	42	M	12
33	Phila.	22	22	M	?
34	Savannah	9	27	S	14
35	Phila.	16	16	S	11
36	Phila.	22	22	M	12
37	Goldsboro	2	18	S	9
38	Pa.	22	22	M	?
39	Phila.	35	35	Sep.	?
40	Phila.	21	22	M	12
41	Phila.	25	25	M	8
42	Phila.	28	28	M	12
43	Ala.	6	17	M	?
44	Phila.	22	22	C. U.	12
45	Phila.	16	16	S	9
46	Phila.	29	29	S	9

47	N. C.	?	30	M	?
48	Phila.	21	21	M	12
49	Phila.	20	20	M	10
50	S. C.	9	29	M	11

Totals:

Composition of Informant's Household											
M	F	H	BF	Z	B	S	D	Other	Total	Fin. Aid	Child Care
1				5	5	1		1	14	DPA	Primipara
						3			4	DPA	M, GM, F
1	1			1	4		1		9	MIC	Primipara
		1					1		3	DPA	Primipara
1	1				4		1		8		Primipara
		1				3	3		8		?
1		1				1	1		5	DPA-MIC	M-in-Law
		1					1		3	MIC	Primipara
		1				1	5		8	DPA-MIC	Sister
		1					2		4	DPA	GM
		1					3		5	MIC	M
							1		2		M's Z (NYD)
			1			2	1	5	10	Soc. Sec.	Z
						2	2		5	DPA	Z
		1				1	3		6	MIC	M-in-Law
1	1					1		4	4	(Unreg.)	Primipara
		1		1		1	2		6	Pennsy.	Z & Z-in-Law
			1			1	1	1	5	MIC	M
1		1				1			4	MIC	M
					1	2	3		7	DPA-MIC	Half-B
								1	2	DPA	Adoption Case
1						2			4	DPA	M
		1				4			6	DPA	Ds (teenage)
		1				2			4	DPA	Girlfriend
						3	2		6	DPA	M
1			1			2			5	Unreg.	BF's M
						1	1		3	DPA	?
1	1				2		1		6	DPA	Primipara
			1				3		5	DPA	Z
			1			3	3		8	DPA-MIC	M
						2	1		4	DPA-MIC	BF's M
		1				3	5		10	Soc. Sec.	H & Ds
		1				4			6	DPA	M
						1	1		3	DPA	Paid Sitter
1				2	2		1	2	9	DPA	Primipara
		1					3		5	Pennsy.	M-in-Law
1				2	2	2	1		9	DPA	M

1		1				1	2		6	DPA	M
						6	6		13	DPA	M
		1				1	3		6	MIC	H
	1	1					1		4		Primipara
		1				2			4	MIC	M
		1				1			3	MIC	? (NYD)
			1			1			3		Primipara
1						1	1		5	DPA	M
						4	7		12		D (teenage)
		1				2	2		6	Union	?
		1				1			3	DPA-MIC	Primipara
		1				3	1		6	DPA	H's B's wife
1		1				3	5		11	DPA-MIC	Neighbor
14	5	24	6	12	20	75	81	10	297		